Stories Celebrating Group Work: It's Not Always Easy to Sit on Your Mouth

Stories Celebrating Group Work: It's Not Always Easy to Sit on Your Mouth has been co-published simultaneously as *Social Work with Groups*, Volume 25, Numbers 1/2 2002.

The *Social Work with Groups* Monographic "Separates"

Below is a list of "separates," which in serials librarianship means a special issue simultaneously published as a special journal issue or double-issue *and* as a "separate" hardbound monograph. (This is a format which we also call a "DocuSerial.")

"Separates" are published because specialized libraries or professionals may wish to purchase a specific thematic issue by itself in a format which can be separately cataloged and shelved, as opposed to purchasing the journal on an on-going basis. Faculty members may also more easily consider a "separate" for classroom adoption.

"Separates" are carefully classified separately with the major book jobbers so that the journal tie-in can be noted on new book order slips to avoid duplicate purchasing.

You may wish to visit Haworth's Website at . . .

http://www.HaworthPress.com

. . . to search our online catalog for complete tables of contents of these separates and related publications.

You may also call 1-800-HAWORTH (outside US/Canada: 607-722-5857), or Fax 1-800-895-0582 (outside US/Canada: 607-771-0012), or e-mail at:

getinfo@haworthpressinc.com

Stories Celebrating Group Work: It's Not Always Easy to Sit on Your Mouth, edited by Roselle Kurland, PhD, and Andrew Malekoff, ACSW (Vol. 25, No. 1/2, 2002). *"A rare glimpse at some of the crucial moments that have inspired, influenced, and created real groupworkers." (Lainey Collins, CSW, Camp Director, The Fresh Air Fund)*

Support Groups: Current Perspectives on Theory and Practice, edited by Maeda J. Galinsky, PhD, and Janice H. Schopler, PhD (Vol. 18, No. 1, 1996). *"Provides a framework for understanding and examining supportive group interventions. Provides descriptions of different kinds of support groups and alerts practioners and educators to issues of planning, implementing, and evaluating such services." (The Brown University Child and Adolescent Behavior Newsletter)*

Social Work with Groups: Expanding Horizons, edited by Stanley Wenocur, PhD, Thomas Vassil, PhD, Paul Ephross, PhD, and Raju Varghese, EdD, MPH (Vol. 16, No. 1/2, 1993). *"Fascinating and interesting. The chapters are excellent, spanning theory and direct practice with groups. . . . Helpful to practitioners and educators. I recommend it highly to both." (Joan K. Parry, DSW, LCSW, Professor, College of Social Work, San Jose State University)*

Group Work Reaching Out: People, Places, and Power, edited by James A. Garland, AB, MSSS (Vol. 15, No. 2/3, 1993). *"Experienced leaders in practice and teaching of social work with groups address the problems and potential of a wide variety of vulnerable, alienated, underserved and politically disenfranchised populations. . . . A must." (Social Work with Groups Newsletter)*

Social Action in Group Work, edited by Abe Vinik and Morris Levin (Vol. 14, No. 3/4, 1992). *"Focuses on getting rid of the causes of problems through group action. . . . Numerous examples are provided for students, educators, researchers, and practitioners." (Social Work with Groups Newsletter)*

Groupwork with Suburbia's Children: Difference, Acceptance, and Belonging, edited by Andrew Malekoff, MSW (Vol 14, No. 1, 1991). *"Provide[s] a careful, professional look into the multiple problems of the children and youth outside of the inner city and minority areas in which we traditionally expect to find such problems." (Social Work with Groups Newsletter)*

Ethnicity and Biculturalism: Emerging Perspectives of Social Group Work, edited by Kenneth L. Chau, PhD (Vol. 13, No. 4, 1991). *"Offers a tremendous help in focusing on the issues and addresses them in a straightforward manner. It is highly recommended for those in 'helping' professions." (Multiculture Publishers Exchange Newsletter)*

Theory and Practice in Social Group Work: Creative Connections, edited by Marie Weil, DSW, Kenneth L. Chau, PhD, and Dannia Southerland, MSW (Supplement #4, 1991). *Here is an important look at creative ways to successfully blend theoretical knowledge with skillful intervention in social group work.* Theory and Practice in Social Group Work *represents leading works in conceptual development that creatively connect practice with theory and also reflect the current diversity of interventions in group work practice.*

Group Work with the Emotionally Disabled, edited by Baruch Levine, PhD (Vol. 13, No. 1, 1990) *"Provides an excellent overview of group work within a variety of settings and with a variety of populations." (Adult Residential Care Journal)*

Groups in Health Care Settings, edited by Janice H. Schopler, PhD, and Maeda J. Galinsky, PhD (Vol. 12, No. 4, 1990). *"This timely collection offers a broad ranging view of what's happening through groups in hospitals and community agencies " (Ruth R. Middleman, EdD, ACSW, Professor, Kent School of Social Work, University of Louisville)*

Roots and New Frontiers in Social Group Work, by Marcus Leiderman, MSW, Martin L. Birnbaum, PhD, and Barbara Dazzo, PhD (Supplement #3, 1989). *"The vitality of contemporary social group work is reflected in this book. . . . A worthwhile contribution to the literature." (Social Work)*

Social Work with Multi-Family Groups, edited by D. Rosemary Cassano, PhD, MSW (Vol. 12, No. 1, 1989). *Better understand the interrelatedness of the primary family group and the formed therapeutic group with this book.*

Group Work with the Poor and Oppressed, edited by Judith A. B. Lee, DSW (Vol. 11, No. 4, 1989). *"A rich source of reference material for those looking for historical, theoretical, and practical references." (Australian Social Work)*

Violence: Prevention and Treatment in Groups, edited by George S. Getzel, DSW (Vol. 11, No. 3, 1989). *"A useful supplement for a library serving a social work, mental health, or family therapy curriculum." (Academic Library Book Review)*

Social Group Work: Competence and Values in Practice, edited by Joseph Lassner, PhD, MSW, Kathleen Powell, MSW, and Elaine Finnegan, MSW (Supplement #2, 1987). *Detailed information on group work theory, group structure, gender and race issues in group work, group work in health care settings, and the use of groups for coping with family issues that will be invaluable for all professionals in their daily practice.*

Working Effectively with Administrative Groups, edited by Ronald W. Toseland, PhD, and Paul H. Ephross, PhD (Vol. 10, No. 2, 1987). *Exciting suggestions for making administrative groups more effective.*

Collectivity in Social Group Work: Concept and Practice, edited by Norma C. Lang, PhD, and Joanne Sulman, MSW (Vol. 9, No. 4, 1987). *A concise and comprehensive examination of the theory of collectivity in social group work.*

Research in Social Group Work, edited by Sheldon D. Rose, PhD, and Ronald A. Feldman (Vol. 9, No. 3, 1987). *Reflects not on only the important advances and strengths in group work research but also some of the deficiencies and gaps that characterize contemporary research in the field.*

The Legacy of William Schwartz: Group Practice as Shared Interaction, edited by Alex Gitterman, EdD, MSW, and Lawrence Schulman (Vol. 8, No. 4, 1986). *This fine volume celebrates William Schwartz's lasting contribution to teaching and scholarship and conveys the power of his ideas and their relevance to contemporary practice.*

Innovations in Social Group Work: Feedback from Practice to Theory, edited by Marvin Parnes, MSW (Supplement #1, 1986). *This classic volume illustrates just how vigorous and inventive social groupwork can be.*

Time as a Factor in Groupwork: Time-Limited Group Experiences, edited by Albert S. Alissi, DSW and Max Casper (Vol. 8, No. 2, 1985). *This informative book provides the helping professional with valuable information on the benefits and drawbacks of time-limited social groupwork.*

Groupwork with Children and Adolescents, edited by Ralph L. Kolodny, MA, MSSS, and James A. Garland, ACSW (Vol. 7, No. 4, 1985). *"Integrates time-tested models and procedures with* *emerging theories and models in a field where a paucity of material exists. . . . Should be of considerable interest to educators as well as social workers." (Voice of Youth Advocates)*

Ethnicity in Social Group Work Practice, edited by Larry E. Davis (Vol. 7, No. 3, 1984). *"Excellent resource. . . . Will serve as a good supplemental text in a generic social group work course or as a main text in a specialized course." (Howard J. Doueck, Social Work Department, State University of New York at Buffalo)*

Groupwork with Women/Groupwork with Men: An Overview of Gender Issues in Social Groupwork Practice, edited by Beth Glover Reed, PhD, and Charles D. Garvin, PhD (Vol. 6, No. 3/4, 1983). *"A variety of approaches to gender-sensitive group work, as well as applications of specific techniques in groups." (Social Work Reporter)*

Activities and Action in Groupwork, edited by Ruth Middleman, EdD, MSW (Vol. 6, No. 1, 1983). *A very helpful resource on the use of activities in social groupwork with a variety of populations.*

The Use of Group Services in Permanency Planning for Children, edited by Sylvia K. Morris, MSW (Vol. 5, No. 4, 1983). *This important sourcebook examines the use of social group work in establishing out-of-home children in permanent homes in an age of federal cutbacks.*

Groupwork with the Frail Elderly, edited by Shura Saul, EdD, CSW (Vol. 5, No. 2, 1983). *"A rich mixture of different types of groups for frail elderly, and for those working with the frail elderly. . . . A valuable aid to social workers, nurses, or any professional working with such groups of individuals." (Journal of Gerontological Nursing)*

Social Groupwork and Alcoholism, edited by Marjorie Altman and Ruth Crocker (Vol. 5, No. 1, 1985). *"Useful information about a number of different kinds of groups in the treatment of alcoholism." (International Journal of Group Psychotherapy)*

Co-Leadership in Social Work with Groups, edited by Catherine P. Papell, DSW and Beulah Rothman, DSW (Vol. 3, No. 4, 1981) *Explores the co-leadership phenomenon in the experience of social work students studying groupwork.*

Stories Celebrating Group Work: It's Not Always Easy to Sit on Your Mouth

Roselle Kurland, PhD
Andrew Malekoff, MSW
Editors

Stories Celebrating Group Work: It's Not Always Easy to Sit on Your Mouth has been co-published simultaneously as *Social Work with Groups*, Volume 25, Numbers 1/2 2002.

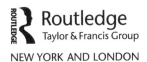

Routledge
Taylor & Francis Group

NEW YORK AND LONDON

First Published by

The Haworth Social Work Practice Press, 10 Alice Street, Binghamton, NY 13904-1580 USA

The Haworth Social Work Practice Press is an imprint of The Haworth Press, Inc., 10 Alice Street, Binghamton, NY 13904-1580 USA.

Published by Routledge
711 Third Avenue, New York, NY 10017
2 Park Square, Milton Park, Abingdon, Oxon, OX14 4RN

Stories Celebrating Group Work: It's Not Always Easy to Sit on Your Mouth has been co-published simultaneously as *Social Work with Groups,* Volume 25, Numbers 1/2 2002.

The development, preparation, and publication of this work has been undertaken with great care. However, the publisher, employees, editors, and agents of The Haworth Press and all imprints of The Haworth Press, Inc., including The Haworth Medical Press® and The Pharmaceutical Products Press®, are not responsible for any errors contained herein or for consequences that may ensue from use of materials or information contained in this work. Opinions expressed by the author(s) are not necessarily those of The Haworth Press, Inc.

Cover illustration © Apollon Menard Used with permission.

Cover design by Lora Wiggins.

Library of Congress Cataloging-in-Publication Data

Stories celebrating group work: it's not always easy to sit on your mouth / edited by Roselle Kurland, and Andrew Malekoff.
     p. cm.
     "Has been co-published simultaneously as Social work with groups, volume 25, numbers 1/2, 2002."
     Includes bibliographical references.
     ISBN 0-7890-1746-6 (hard : alk. paper) -- ISBN 0-7890-1747-4 (pbk: alk. paper)
     1. Social group work–Case studies. I. Kurland, Roselle. II. Malekoff, Andrew. III. Social work with groups (Haworth Press)
HV45 .S83 2002
361.4–dc21   2002152089

Publisher's Note
The publisher has gone to great lengths to ensure the quality of this reprint
but points out that some imperfections in the original may be apparent.

ABOUT THE EDITORS

Roselle Kurland, PhD, is Professor at the Hunter College School of Social Work. She is the author (with Helen Northen) of the third edition of the text *Social Work with Groups,* and (with Robert Salmon) of *Teaching a Methods Course in Social Work with Groups.* Dr. Kurland has written and presented many papers on group work theory, practice, and education, and has done consultation and training with a wide range of social work agencies and organizations.

Andrew Malekoff, MSW, is Associate Executive Director for the North Shore Child and Family Guidance Center in Roslyn Heights, New York. He is also Adjunct Professor of Social Work at Adelphi University, a widely published author, and internationally known lecturer. The most recent of his three books is the critically acclaimed *Group Work with Adolescents: Principles and Practice.*

Stories Celebrating Group Work: It's Not Always Easy to Sit on Your Mouth

CONTENTS

About the Contributors

Ann Rosegrant Alvarez, MSW, PhD, is Associate Professor, School of Social Work, Wayne State University, 137 Thompson Home, 4756 Cass Avenue, Detroit, MI.

Toby Berman-Rossi, MSW, DSW, is Professor, Barry University School of Social Work 11300 NE Second Avenue, Miami Shores, FL.

Mary C. Bitel, MSW, is Director of Girls' Programs, Interfaith Neighbors, 14 East 109 Street, New York, NY.

Margot Breton, MSW, is Professor, Emerita, Faculty of Social Work, University of Toronto, 160 Rosedale Heights Drive, Toronto, Ontario.

Cynthia G. Cavallo, MA, is Executive Director, Coalition on Child Abuse and Neglect, 229 Seventh Street, Garden City, NY.

Marcia B. Cohen, MSSW, PhD, is Professor, University of New England School of Social Work, 716 Stevens Avenue, Portland, ME.

Roseline Felix, MSW, is Coordinator of Haitian Family Life Program, North Shore Child and Family Guidance Center, 147 Renken Boulevard, Franklin Square, NY.

Alex Gitterman, MSW, EdD, is Professor, University of Connecticut School of Social Work, 1798 Asylum Avenue, West Hartford, CT.

Roselle Kurland, MSW, PhD, is Professor, Hunter College School of Social Work, 129 East 79 Street, New York, NY.

Marion S. Levine, MSW, is Executive Director, North Shore Child and Family Guidance Center, 480 Old Westbury Road, Roslyn Heights, NY.

Andrew Malekoff, MSW, is Associate Director, North Shore Child and Family Guidance Center, 480 Old Westbury Road, Roslyn Heights, NY.

Flavio Francisco Marsiglia, MSW, PhD, is Associate Professor, Arizona State University School of Social Work, P.O. Box 873711, Tempe, AZ.

Rachel Miller, MSW, is Senior Social Worker, North Shore-Long Island Jewish Health System, Hillside Hospital, Research Department, 75-59 263 Street, Glen Oaks, NY.

Emily Wolff Newmann, MSW, is Coordinator, Dream House Program, Jewish Family and Children's Services, 364 Precita Avenue, San Francisco, CA.

Helen Northen, MSW, PhD, is Distinguished Professor Emerita, University of Southern California, 1942 Westlake Avenue, #2316, Seattle, WA.

Anna Nosko, MSW, is Social Worker, Family Services Association of Toronto, 8 Taber Road, Toronto, Ontario, Canada.

Catherine P. Papell, MSW, DSW, is Professor Emerita, Adelphi University School of Social Work, 146-18 Cherry Avenue, Flushing, NY.

Camille P. Roman, MSW, is Private Practitioner and Adjunct Associate Professor, Hunter College School of Social Work, 970 Park Avenue, New York, NY.

Linda Yael Schiller, MSW, LICSW, is Adjunct Assistant Professor, Boston University School of Social Work, Private Clinical Practice, 98 Channing Road, Watertown, MA.

Lawrence Shulman, MSW, EdD, is Dean, School of Social Work, University at Buffalo, 685 Baldy Hall, Buffalo, NY.

Dominique Moyse Steinberg, MSW, is Adjunct Faculty, Smith College School for Social Work, Northampton, MA.

Michael W. Wagner, MSW, is Intake Supervisor/Coordinator of Foster Parent Training and Development, The Children's Aid Society, 61 Lafayette Road, Tappan, NY.

Whitney Wright, MSW, is Director of Youth CAN LINC-Project Impact, Bayview Hunter's Point Foundation, 2758 22nd Street, San Francisco, CA.

Introduction

Roselle Kurland
Andrew Malekoff

This special publication celebrates the 25th anniversary of *Social Work with Groups*. In the Spring of 1978, in the Journal's first issue (1: 1), Catherine Papell and Beulah Rothman, the founding editors, articulated an editorial policy that continues today. They wanted the journal to

> serve as a vehicle of communication for the several sectors of our profession wherein the small group heritage and the building of knowledge and skills of group practice are embodied. There are those who represent the early group work tradition from the community and neighborhood centers with focus on socialization in groups and the contribution of the healthy group to social betterment. There are those who represent the clinical tradition with focus on the therapeutic value of the small group and on the family as a small group. There are those who represent the community and planning tradition with focus on mobilizing and developing social resources and neighborhoods through the energies of task groups. Finally, there are those who represent administration and social policy with focus on welding together a humanizing service system through the collective efforts of staff and community groups. It is to the enrichment and dissemination of these professional labors that this journal of group theory and practice is dedicated.

[Haworth co-indexing entry note]: "Introduction." Roselle Kurland, and Andrew Malekoff. Co-published simultaneously in *Social Work with Groups* (The Haworth Social Work Practice Press, an imprint of The Haworth Press, Inc.) Vol. 25, No. 1/2, 2002, pp. 1-7; and: *Stories Celebrating Group Work: It's Not Always Easy to Sit on Your Mouth* (ed: Roselle Kurland, and Andrew Malekoff) The Haworth Social Work Practice Press, an imprint of The Haworth Press, Inc., 2002, pp. 1-7. Single or multiple copies of this article are available for a fee from The Haworth Document Delivery Service [1-800-HAWORTH, 9:00 a.m. - 5:00 p.m. (EST). E-mail address: getinfo@haworthpressinc.com].

1

In the quarter century of its existence, this Journal has been important in the development of the theory and practice of social work with groups. It has provided a vital place where those in our profession who have particular interest in and commitment to group work practice can feel at home, have a sense of belonging and an outlet to discuss their own interests and to read about those of colleagues. The Journal has helped to create a sense of community among group workers.

The 25th anniversary volume needed to be special. To make it so, we asked a range of social workers–young and old, practitioners and teachers, "famous" and not-so-famous–each to write a personal narrative addressing a specific theme about which we thought they would have particular expertise and interest. Each author was asked to tell a story about the evolution of his/her understanding, appreciation, and skill in that area. The result is a unique collection of stories, simultaneously enjoyable and educational.

This volume also marks our tenth year together as editors. Our partnership is unique: the pairing of one person who is primarily a social work educator and one who is primarily a social work practitioner. We have tried to continue to establish the excellence of this Journal. Through our correspondence and work with new writers, practitioners in particular, and through workshops on writing that we have led at a number of Symposia of the Association for the Advancement of Social Work With Groups, we have tried to encourage new authors to write about their ideas and practice. Our aim has been to have the Journal be a place that invites thoughtful exploration and examination of ideas.

Throughout our tenure, the editorials in the Journal have been an expression of ideas about the trends and needs that we see reflected in our profession. Frankly, there have been times when we wondered whether these editorials were being read or whether readers simply went immediately to the articles that interested them in each issue. Every once in a while, though, someone would comment to us about an idea expressed in a particular editorial and we would take heart. Our editorials do provide a representation of some of the issues and trends in group work of the past ten years, and we take the occasion of this special publication as an opportunity to review some of those that we consider particularly important.

WORKING TOGETHER

First, some insight on how we work together from a 1998 editorial (21: 1/2). As editors we get together, in between extended phone conversations several times a year to do the work of the Journal. One of us (Kurland) teaches at a university and the other (Malekoff) practices at a mental health center. When we meet, our discussions about the direction of the journal and about individual articles under consideration shift back and forth between the classroom and the field. We have tried to shape the journal to appeal to practitioners, educators and students by bringing together the conceptual and the practical.

Before assuming our editorial roles we had not worked together or even met one another. In the early days of our joint editorship we spent time getting acquainted and figuring out whether and how we might work together. There were the nuts and bolts decisions, such as where we would meet and who would handle what correspondence. For example, after a few trips to each of our host settings we agreed to centralize operations and meet at Hunter College School of Social Work. This meant that one of us (Malekoff) would take the Long Island Railroad into New York City for meetings. One of the tradeoffs for his travel expenses was lunch to be provided by Kurland at the greasy spoon around the corner from the College on Lexington Avenue.

There were also more complex decisions, such as whether our editorials should be summary previews of each issue's content or opinion pieces and reflections related to contemporary issues and trends. We chose the latter. We gradually discovered that, while we do not always agree, we speak the same language when it comes to group work. This was far from a given at the beginning when we were strangers.

CHOOSING ISSUES TO WRITE ABOUT

Looking back over ten years, we discovered that the issues we chose to write about fit into a few categories: writing guidelines and suggestions, exploring group work's role in social issues and trends (e.g., managed care, after school programs, addressing violence), the state of group work education, emphasizing selected practice issues (use of activities, the over-use of curriculum-driven groups, involuntary clients, group composition, dealing with silence), life shattering events (terrorist attacks of September 11th, 2001), and how we as group workers take care of ourselves.

ENCOURAGING ASPIRING WRITERS

One of our favorite themes has been to encourage people to write, especially beginning writers and practitioners. In our second editorial in 1992 (15: 4), we offered suggestions for aspiring writers. What we would like to see in *Social Work with Groups,* we wrote, are articles that bring together the doing and thinking of group work practice. In articles that emphasize knowledge of the needs of a particular population, implications for and illustrations of group work practice based on such knowledge need to be integral. In articles that portray practice through the presentation of descriptive vignettes and examples, the rationale that underpins the practice, the thinking behind it, and the implications for future practice with groups are crucial elements. In short, our mantra for writers to the journal has become: *Punctuate descriptive articles with concepts and bring conceptual articles to life with illustrations.*

LOSING OUR WAY

One of the most frustrating themes we wrote about is how our profession seems to be losing its way. In a 2001 editorial (23: 4) we remarked on the growing emphasis on research in doctoral programs and noted that, historically, practice has been at the heart of social work. To learn to work with people skillfully and with understanding remains the primary reason that people enter the profession. Research can certainly contribute to that goal. It plays an important role in doing so. But it seems to us that research is becoming an end in itself. If the primary aim of doctoral programs is to turn out skillful researchers who can compete with other disciplines for status, prove that social work interventions work, and enhance social work's prestige, then it is not surprising that such programs are having difficulty. Those are not the reasons that most social workers would be interested in seeking doctoral education. Current trends seem to be devaluing quality practice. We need to reverse that direction. We are in danger of losing our profession if we do not.

SEPTEMBER 11TH, 2001

The role of group work in the aftermath of life shattering events is not a choice that we as editors make to write about. We consider it a duty. Following the terrorist attacks of September 11th, both of us, in our own way, used our practice skills in the classroom and field to help students and colleagues and survivors and mourners to debrief and defuse in the aftermath of the most horrific event of our lifetime.

The first editorial we wrote following 9/11 was a narrative account of front-line group work by one of us (Malekoff), preceded by an introduction by the other (24: 3/4). The emphasis in the narrative was on a lesson learned, "I learned that trauma isolates. I know that group work connects." The core qualities of a group worker are emphasized–the need to be flexible, to be willing to switch gears and throw one's original plans and content out the window when a different approach and different content are needed.

Among the uncertainties that we confront in today's volatile world, what is certain is that groups and the connections among people that they can foster continue to be important and much needed.

TAKING CARE OF OURSELVES

One of our favorite editorials was written in 1995. It is about the need for group workers to take care of themselves and one another (18: 4). We conclude with our sentiment on the subject.

How do we take care of ourselves? When you've finished a particularly difficult group meeting in which you are left reeling and dazed, what helps? Or what about a meeting in which you are left feeling deeply moved and you know you have just been a part of something special? Is your colleague in the next room or down the hall or a phone call away someone whom you are eager to see and share with? Or do you flinch at the thought? Does the place in which you spend the better part of your day, and maybe evening, invite collegial support?

How do we take care of ourselves? What we know about groups is relevant here. *First,* we know that people are social beings who need the affirmation and support of others. *Second,* we know that a good group is one where members can really be themselves and be accepted by the other group members, that in a good group there is no need to put on airs or to pretend to be someone one is not in order to gain the acceptance of one's peers. *Third,* we know that in a group attention must be paid simultaneously to the total group and to each of the individual group members.

How do we take care of ourselves? Such basic principles apply. We all need affirmation, support and understanding from at least some of our colleagues. We need to be able to be ourselves with those colleagues and to know that we will be accepted by them, even when we may disagree about particular approaches or points of view.

And, of course, there are times when we are nourished by solitude, when we take the time to think things through on our own. Such moments can generate creative expression, expression for no reason but to satisfy one's soul. Music, art, writing or whatever activities we use to tap the spirit in our groups can work for us as individual workers as well. Such moments of solitude are valued, especially when one is solid in the knowledge that one also "belongs" to a "good group" of colleagues.

How do we take care of ourselves? We need to seek out and then value true colleagues–those who will listen, understand, share, accept, challenge, affirm, validate, support, disagree, respect. Such persons are rare. Too often, those with whom we work tend not to really listen or hear or understand, but rather to compete. Too often the stories and experiences we share with others become too quickly the bases of their comparisons: "Oh that's nothing. You should have seen what happened in my group . . ." Or the patronizingly dismissive, "Been there, done that." Or they become the jumping off points for premature and unwanted, unsought advice: "You should have done this . . ." or "Did you try that . . ."

True colleagues are, indeed, rare. We need them. We need to seek them out. And when we find them, we need to treasure them. And in the work that we do, that is so very demanding, difficult, moving and special, we also need to be real colleagues to others.

This special *Silver Anniversary* volume is offered with a collegial spirit. We hope that the personal stories that follow will leave you moved, tickled, inspired, educated, and . . . supported.

Memories of *Social Work with Groups:* Volume 1 (1978) Through Volume 14 (1991)

Catherine P. Papell

Reminiscing on these fourteen years is both exhilarating and painful, exhilarating because the task of co-editorship of *Social Work with Groups* represented an essential professional involvement in my life, and painful because it was the ending of a joint endeavor with my beloved colleague and friend, Beulah Rothman.

In the beginning, 1978, we were asked by Bill Cohen, publisher of The Haworth Press, Inc., to edit a journal concerned with the group method in the profession of Social Work. Neither of us knew anything about editing a journal, but we loved our memories of practice in group work agencies and we loved teaching social group work in the MSW curriculum and writing about it. We sat down and began to compose an Editorial Policy Statement, conveying our understanding of social group work as an inherent part of the profession of social work. I repeat the Editorial Policy Statement in full since it has been affirmed again and again throughout the twenty-five years of the journal's existence:

THE EDITORIAL POLICY STATEMENT 1978

There is no profession that places a greater value on the individual in his social context than does the profession of social work. For most people the social context becomes manageable and definable

[Haworth co-indexing entry note]: "Memories of *Social Work with Groups:* Volume 1 (1978) Through Volume 14 (1991)." Papell, Catherine P. Co-published simultaneously in *Social Work with Groups* (The Haworth Social Work Practice Press, an imprint of The Haworth Press, Inc.) Vol. 25, No. 1/2, 2002, pp. 9-13; and: *Stories Celebrating Group Work: It's Not Always Easy to Sit on Your Mouth* (ed: Roselle Kurland, and Andrew Malekoff) The Haworth Social Work Practice Press, an imprint of The Haworth Press, Inc., 2002, pp. 9-13. Single or multiple copies of this article are available for a fee from The Haworth Document Delivery Service [1-800-HAWORTH, 9:00 a.m. - 5:00 p.m. (EST). E-mail address: getinfo@haworthpressinc.com].

through the small group. Now more than ever, in an alienating and anomic world, there is the necessity for the human group to carry its functions: the linking of individuals with each other as they struggle to achieve fullness and the production of morale, leadership, and cooperation, the bonding ingredients for a viable society.

During the past two decades as the profession has been strengthening its central unity it has seemed that the unique social work contribution to understanding and working with the small group was being lost. It is our conviction, to the contrary, that in this period of time social work has been quietly developing a new and mature identity in relation to group practice. This journal hopes to set forth that new identity, incorporating the vitality of our history with the richness and complexity of the psychosocial orientation of our profession. It is no longer only the group workers in the social work profession who carry the passion for the human group and the commitment to its use in relation to social work purposes, but the profession itself.

It is the intent of *Social Work with Groups* to serve as a vehicle of communication for the several sectors of our profession wherein the small group heritage and the building of knowledge and skills of group practice are embodied. There are those who represent the early group work tradition from the community and neighborhood centers with focus on socialization in groups and the contribution of the healthy group to social betterment. There are those who represent the clinical tradition with focus on the therapeutic value of the small group and on the family as a small group. There are those who represent the community and planning tradition with focus on mobilizing and developing social resources and neighborhoods through the energies of task groups. Finally, there are those who represent administration and social policy with focus on welding together a humanizing service system through the collective efforts of staff and community groups. It is to the enrichment and dissemination of those professional labors that this journal of group work theory and practice is dedicated.

In view of the social context of 2001-2: terror, deadly conflict throughout the world, and new levels of diversity in paradoxical relation to uniformity, the Editors, Advisory Board, and readers might undertake to revise The Editorial Policy Statement. I would hope it would not alter the view of group work in the profession of Social Work, but it should address with greater courage and specificity the present and on-going injuries to humanity and the sharpened need for the values and skills of social group work.

I am recalling Social Work's professional issues in 1978. It was the era of methods integration in education for Social Work. Beulah and I had both been active in creating a Foundation Methods course, and teaching and writing about it (Papell, 1978, in K. Dea, Ed., *New Ways of Teaching Social Work Practice,* New York: CSWE). However, we had not intended (it might be called innocence!) that foundation practice would diminish the teaching of group work practice. Indeed, we hoped it would enhance methodological opportunities for service. However, that was not to be. For this reason Beulah and I saw this new journal as vital in highlighting the importance of the teaching of the group work method in the profession's educational system. We both felt very pleased with the name for the journal that we decided on, *Social Work with Groups: A Journal of Community and Clinical Practice.* It said what we both wanted to say in undertaking this task of co-editing a new journal on social group work practice.

In considering "social group work" and "social work with groups," Beulah and I used the terms interchangeably, the one for the breadth of the method within the profession and the other for the depth of its demo-cratic value base. The issue of which term to use seems to illustrate the enormous complexity of the social work profession. We will eternally struggle with the interrelated nature of humankind in social contexts. A social worker cannot erase any dimension from his/her consideration, regardless of wherein lies the compelling focus of the specific task. It is through the ongoing consideration and continuous reconsideration of such complexity that all social workers take into account their profes-sion's societal function. It is a dialectical challenge that never ends.

Leafing through the fourteen volumes that Beulah and I co-edited, I am overwhelmed by the memories of the wonderful authors whose pa-pers were published and with whom we had many lively conversations by letter and phone. Starting with the earliest issues, we had to solicit papers. Group workers were not yet accustomed to writing about their work.

As the journal continued successfully, the flow of papers increased and we no longer sought out authors. However, we did begin, early on, to invite guest editors to prepare an issue on a special subject. Tom Douglas, Senior Lecturer in Social Policy and Social Work, University of Keele, was our first Guest Editor (Vol. 4, No. 1, 1981). He prepared a very impressive volume on Groupwork in Great Britain. We were very pleased with how adventurous we had been in writing to Tom Douglas and proud that we could publish his distinguished paper on theory and those of his British colleagues.

Many special issues followed, each prepared by a social group worker who could elicit a substantive array of papers around the area of group work practice that was his/her expertise.

The range of human concerns about which social group workers wrote in these special issues–and throughout all the fourteen volumes of the journal–illustrate the broad and deep approach to social work with groups that Beulah and I were hoping would be recaptured and revived in the profession of Social Work through the presence of this journal in its literature. It readily appears that there is something precious in the social work profession's social group work method that is historically embedded, and profoundly useful and unique amongst all helping professions whose work takes place in groups.

Beulah and I prepared a special issue on *Education for Social Work with Groups* (Vol. 11, No. 1/2, 1988). We had failed to indicate to The Haworth Press that it should be treated, as were special issues, in an available book form and listed in its *Social Work with Groups* Series. The papers, by a very exemplary group of social work educators, were indeed special. As an example, the late Howard Goldstein wrote a beautiful paper on "A Cognitive-Humanistic/Social Learning Perspective on Social Group Work Practice." Beulah and I were convinced that he had been a group worker in his youth! The Preface for that issue also was important to us, since it was our effort to celebrate ten years of the journal. In the Preface we tried to identify what we felt to be the significant professional enrichment of social group work practice and theory in that decade.

Four times a year for fourteen years Beulah and I wrote the Preface with loving care. Both of us would collect our thoughts based on the articles and book reviews that were to make up the issue. We would then meet together and compose the Preface. Sometimes one or the other of us would have further ideas and we might meet again to finalize it. When Beulah moved to Florida and Barry University, I would travel periodically to work on the current issue. The Prefaces carried a restored vision for group work's sustainability in the societal function of the profession and its continuing contribution toward social justice and the well being of humans.

The full story must be told. . . . In January 1990, Beulah Rothman was diagnosed with lung cancer. The Prefaces in Volume 14, Numbers 1 and 2 both carry this note: "This Volume was prepared and the Foreword written before Beulah Rothman's death in August 1990." The Preface for Volume 14, Number 3/4 was mine to write alone:

> With this issue of *Social Work with Groups*–and with this Editorial–the era of the original and present co-editorship is drawn to a close. Beulah Rothman and I had decided early in the fateful year of her illness and death that we were ready to yield to others the excitement of editing the social group work journal. In April of 1990 we wrote to Bill Cohen, Publisher of The Haworth Press, Inc., resigning as Co-Editors and proposing persons to replace us. Our suggestions were graciously accepted and with the completion of this issue, Number 3/4 of Volume 14, our responsibilities are terminated.
>
> The new Editors are Roselle Kurland, Professor of Social Group Work at Hunter School of Social Work, and Andrew Malekoff, Coordinator of the Suburban Family Life Center and the Alcohol Treatment and Prevention Services at the North Shore Child and Family Guidance Center. Volume 15 (1992) is being prepared by them in their new roles. (p. xii)
>
> For the retiring co-editors of *Social Work with Groups* the journal was a mission! The power of healthy group life for the society, for individual growth and well-being, and as a means of social work helping was a commitment. It remained so throughout Beulah Rothman's life and continues in mine. This has been shared by the members of the journal's Advisory Board during these fourteen years and I believe by you, its readers. The work to be done in such an endeavor cannot ever be complete, so may it go on with new inspiration and vitality in *Social Work with Groups,* in the literature of social group work and of the social work profession! (p. xiv)

And so it has, Roselle and Andy! Congratulations to you on the 25th anniversary of its publication, to its Advisory Board, the Publisher, the journal's authors, AND its readers!

A Tale of Transformation:
How I Became a Group Worker

Marcia B. Cohen

AMBIVALENCE: THE EARLY YEARS

My students think I was born a group worker. I suspect some of my colleagues do too. I have told them otherwise but they forget. Sometimes I forget. The truth is that I began my professional social work career without any group work background or identity. Having made this confession, I will attempt to chronicle the personal/professional journey of discovery that led me to group work.

When I entered a Master's Program in Social Work in the early 1970s, I was a young woman, fresh from the experiences of 1960s social activism, eager to fight for social change. This drew me to community organizing. I enjoyed working with people one on one, however, and had already some of this kind of work as a volunteer. This drew me to social casework. My senior year in college was spent trying to decide between the two. I was barely aware of group work.

Unable to make a decision, I applied to three graduate social work programs as a potential case work student and to three others as a C.O. student. Catholic University, where I ended up, was one of the schools to which I had applied in casework. During student orientation, I heard more about the C.O. concentration and feeling certain this was where I belonged, I made a last minute switch. By December, I realized that while C.O. ideology was dear to my heart, casework practice more

[Haworth co-indexing entry note]: "A Tale of Transformation: How I Became a Group Worker." Cohen, Marcia B. Co-published simultaneously in *Social Work with Groups* (The Haworth Social Work Practice Press, an imprint of The Haworth Press, Inc.) Vol. 25, No. 1/2, 2002, pp. 15-22; and: *Stories Celebrating Group Work: It's Not Always Easy to Sit on Your Mouth* (ed: Roselle Kurland, and Andrew Malekoff) The Haworth Social Work Practice Press, an imprint of The Haworth Press, Inc., 2002, pp. 15-22. Single or multiple copies of this article are available for a fee from The Haworth Document Delivery Service [1-800-HAWORTH, 9:00 a.m. - 5:00 p.m. (EST). E-mail address: getinfo@haworthpressinc.com].

15

closely matched my personal strengths. I tried to switch back but was informed that it was too late, I had missed too much casework content. Undaunted, I researched other options and discovered I could transfer to Columbia, as a casework student, for my second year. I returned to my native New York City. I liked Columbia, but still felt that something was missing. I knew I didn't want to switch back to C.O., but both paths seemed to require a trade off. Casework or community work? Individual change or social change? Why couldn't I do both?

Columbia had a very strong group work presence at the time, so I became much more aware of it than I had been at Catholic. With such notables as Bill Schwartz, Alex Gitterman, and others on the faculty, group work seemed alluring, but I had switched around too many times to consider yet another change. I took enough casework and C.O. courses to fulfill the requirements of each, and as a result missed out on the opportunity to take courses from these group work giants.

I worked in a number of fields of practice following graduation. Working as a medical social worker and later at a shelter for abused women, there were expectations that I facilitate support groups. Just before my very first group work experience, my supervisor handed me a copy of an article by William Schwartz (Schwartz, 1961). The article was great, although some more direct supervision would also have been helpful. I approached this first group with trepidation. No one showed and I was very relieved.

Many groups later, I had gotten over most of my fears and had become reasonably comfortable with the facilitator role. What I lacked in training and supervision, I tried to make up for in observational ability, interpersonal skill, and the belief in the capacity of groups to bring about positive change. I learned a great deal from experience, mostly from making mistakes. My work with groups in domestic violence settings was particularly important in teaching me about the power of groups and the strengths of group members.

AN ABUSED WOMEN'S GROUP

A group for women in abusive relationships, which I facilitated in a domestic violence agency in the early 1980s, illustrates some of the group work principles I learned by the seat of my pants. All members of the group had been in oppressive, violent relationships, tacitly supported by the larger society which privileges men over women. The group was unusual in the extent of its diversity, with members ranging from affluent to very poor, and including Caucasian, African-American, and Latina women.

As different as these women were from each other, their commonalities drew them together. As a group, members examined the ways in which their husbands and boyfriends had controlled, demeaned, and disempowered them, they saw their own experiences reflected in each other's lives and began to see each other and themselves in terms of strengths. The mutuality and connection in this group were powerful and enabled them to analyze their individual and shared oppression in order to better understand and combat it. Years later, when I read Larry Shulman's (1992) discussion of the relationship between a group's ability to handle diversity and its degree of commonality in connection with group purpose, I immediately remembered this group. I finally understood why the women saw each other so completely as "sisters under the skin," despite their considerable differences.

Although the members of this group emphasized their similarities, frequently exclaiming, "Our stories are so much alike, we must have all married the same man!," they also came to acknowledge and appreciate their differences. As the group members drew on each other for mutual aid and learned from each other's experiences, I learned a great deal from them. In addition to gaining awareness about the power of collectivity and the strength of individual group members, I learned about the interconnectedness between diversity, oppression, and role of empowerment and collective action.

GROUP WORK WITH HOMELESS WOMEN

Several years later, while a doctoral student at Brandeis, I was offered a Lecturer position at Columbia, in connection with a special project on homelessness. My primary role was to work as a team leader, developing and supervising a residential program for homeless women. We developed a very group-oriented program, basically learning by trial and error.

It was at this point in my career that my interest in groups took a giant leap forward. Groups had been in my professional background for many years, and my experiences working with them had been positive. Now they were very much part of my foreground. I was busy developing a group program for homeless women who were survivors of the streets and of the worst our mental health system has had to offer. Individually some of the women seemed very crazy, very scary, others were extremely withdrawn, some seemed quite fragile. In our group activities (art, cooking, crafts, recreation, newsletter, movies, current events, exercise, etc.), most of the women emerged as strong and active participants, who grew along with the groups. I was amazed at their transformation.

I will always remember Abby, who initially was not a participant in any of the formed group activities, but was an important member of the larger residential group. When I first met her she seemed catatonic, spending most of her time in a prone position on the living room floor, not bathing, dressing, or caring for herself in any way. She ate food that was placed beside her on the floor by the staff of the residence. Abby's primitive existence was extremely disturbing. I tried to get to know her, but initially met with only limited success. Two years later, after an involuntary hospitalization, medication, and a lot of work on Abby's part, she was very effectively co-facilitating the newsletter group, with one of my social work students. It turned out that Abby was a very bright, educated woman, with many skills and abilities, as well as a history of trauma and pain.

I also developed a Movie Group, in the same residential program, which served as a vehicle for talking about "taboo" subjects, such as mental illness, a current events group which served as a vehicle to raise consciousness about societal issues such as homelessness and poverty, and a dinner group which functioned as a skill and community building group. Some groups were intended primarily to be just for fun, in the historic spirit of group work: an art group, a recreation group, and a dance group. Of course, these groups were rich in opportunities for skill building (for the group members as well as the facilitators).

A GROUP WORKER IS BORN

Meanwhile, although most of my work was with the homeless program, I was a member of the Columbia School of Social Work faculty and teaching one course. I was quickly drawn to and taken under the nurturing wing of the faculty's group work contingent: Alex Gitterman, Renee Solomon, Toby Berman-Rossi, and the late Irving Miller. They taught me about the importance of group work, of the synergistic properties of groups, and of the centrality of mutual aid. They also began to teach me about the culture of group work and its special legacy within the field of social work. I had not previously understood that group work had such distinct values and history, no doubt because I missed taking group work courses as a student.

The influence of these mentors dovetailed with my practice experiences and propelled me toward a group work identity. As much as I had always enjoyed working with groups and had recognized the potential of groups to tap group members' strengths and enhance their power, I was now learning about another aspect of group work which appealed to me greatly.

Throughout my professional career, I struggled with the unhappy perception that my ideological commitment to community work and social action was at odds with my natural abilities, which seemed to be more in the direct practice arena. As in my student days, I continued to question why I should be forced to choose between community practice and direct practice, wishing that I could combine the two in such a way that would maximize my strengths and my beliefs. I will never forget the day I noticed the words on the cover of a borrowed copy of *Social Work with Groups:* "A Journal of Community and Clinical Practice." *Both of them, in one place?* It brought tears to my eyes. I subscribed the same day.

I finally understood why I was so drawn to group work and group workers. Group work offered more than recognizing and harnessing the awesome power of working with people in groups. It offered a way of being a social worker which did not require choosing between fighting for social change and working for individual and interpersonal change. This understanding was a milestone for me in my evolving identity as a group worker at a time when casework was becoming increasingly clinical and community organization was evolving into administration practice, I had finally found a home for myself in social work, someplace in the middle of that micro/macro practice continuum where I could fit in and be a valued member. I had found a group where I belonged.

I was still lacking a group work education, however. I had gleaned some knowledge from colleagues but had not done much of the critical reading, nor had I applied group work theory to my own practice. Fortunately for me, right around that time, Toby Berman-Rossi was looking for someone to co-author an article on homelessness and group work, for a special issue of SWWG. She approached me with this idea, assuring me that she would compensate for any gaps there might be in my group work knowledge if I would provide the data on the group practice. Little did I know that compensating for gaps in my knowledge would mean seeing to it that I filled them in! In place of the group work education I had missed at Columbia in the 1970s, I had an extensive and rigorous independent study in group work from Professor Berman-Rossi in the 1980s. After providing me with extensive readings, and spending hours discussing group development, group process, mutual aid, and the role of the worker with me, Toby and I began to analyze my students' process recordings of the Dinner Group. Toby helped me see how often the group worker, either myself or a student supervised by me (the group lasted more than 5 years and facilitators changed over time), inadvertently sabotaged the group's development. I was aghast but grateful to learn how an understanding of the principles of group development could have helped the facilitators promote group development, rather than creating obstacles to the group's growth. As we described it (Berman-Rossi and Cohen, 1989):

> The workers found it necessary to make critical decisions for the group. Once Teresa arrived late and her task had been completed by another member. She refused to clean and had to be asked to leave the group. When Bella insisted on making the spaghetti an hour early, the workers had to take the spaghetti away. The members were told that the workers would have the final say over what goes on in the group. There were no immediate reactions and the workers didn't reach for any. . . . Tensions over food and task assignments continued. Arguments came to physical blows. While the members were severely critical of each other, they hardly ever directly challenged the workers. (p. 71)

The fact that the Dinner Group did grow and progress over time, despite the limitations in knowledge on the part of the group facilitators, is a testament to the inherent nature of groups to grow and thrive, even in the face of challenges and constraints. As we concluded in the article:

> The members' reconciling of the workers' power took place over the life of the group. Viewing the group over five years tells the story of how these women eventually became strengthened to assert their independence from the workers. The eventual shift to a sharing of power was based on the recognition that not only were the members competent to handle group issues, but they were indeed theirs to handle. It was their group, just as the original workers had hoped it would be. (Berman-Rossi and Cohen, 1989, p. 75)

AND THE WORK CONTINUES

By the 1990s, I had moved to my present teaching job in Maine where I teach and write articles on group work, and work with groups of homeless people and psychiatric survivors in the community. I also became very active in the Association for the Advancement of Social Work With Groups (AASWG). It was at a 1994 AASWG symposium in Hartford that I first met Audrey Mullender, an author from the U.K. whose work on social action group work (Mullender and Ward, 1991) had impressed me greatly. Audrey and I began a conversation about bridging individual and social change goals in action group work that lasted through two more symposia, San Diego in 1995 and Ann Arbor in 1996. I finally suggested we write together.

Our article, "The Personal in the Political: Exploring the Group Work Continuum from Individual to Social Change Goals" (Cohen and Mullender, 1999) explores many of the themes I had been struggling with 25 years earlier, particularly the false dichotomy between social change and individual change. After examining several different groups, we concluded that:

> What (this) means is that rather than the familiar continuum of three mutually exclusive levels of operation: *personal, interpersonal, and social*, we might better reflect the complex world of practice if we think in terms of all groups having individual content, most groups utilizing and valuing mutually supportive interactional content, but some groups reaching out beyond their own boundaries towards an external social change focus . . . Social action groups . . . can potentially span the entire continuum of levels of operation, from the intensely personal to the outwardly political. (p. 25-26)

Indeed, I believe that all groups can change, evolve, mutate and grow as they develop over time and as needs arise. For example, an activist poor people's group I am currently working with, recently set aside a previously planned agenda of strategizing the logistics of mobilizing a protest at city hall, in order to address the needs and fears of a new member who was on the verge of eviction and had come to the group for support. These group members never questioned the wisdom of moving back and forth between personal, interpersonal, and social change goals. It never occurred to them that they might be mutually exclusive or that they had to choose. The new member was able to use the information gained from the group to avoid eviction, at least temporarily, and the city hall protest was a big success.

Groups are truly places where individual change and social change can co-exist and enrich each other, particularly when mutual aid is present to serve as the glue that holds the group together. It may have taken me a while to come to this understanding, but I cherish the discoveries I have had along the way.

REFERENCES

Berman-Rossi, Toby and Cohen, Marcia B. (1989). Group development and shared decision making: Working with homeless mentally ill women. *Social Work with Groups*, 11 (4), 63-78.

Cohen, Marcia B. and Mullender, Audrey (1999). The Personal in the Political: Exploring the Group Work Continuum from Individual to Social Change Goals, *Social Work with Groups*, 22 (1), 13-31.

Mullender, Audrey and Ward, David (1991). Empowerment through social action group work: The "self-directed" approach, *Social Work with Groups*, 14 (3/4), 125-139.

Schwartz. William (1961). The social worker in the group, In *New Perspectives on Services to Groups: Theory, Organization, Practice*, New York: NASW, 7-34.

Shulman, Lawrence (1992). *The Skills of Helping Individuals Families and Groups.* Itasca, IL: Peacock Publishers.

A Rewarding Group Worker's Journey

Margot Breton

On a sunny morning in October 1986, I was sitting at a café on the main *piazza* of Perugia, a beautiful hilltown north of Rome. I was playing hooky from teaching at the University of Toronto, having accompanied my husband, who was planning a conference with fellow economists. He had brought along a book by Leonardo Boff, the Brazilian liberation theologian. I, being a social worker and no doubt feeling somewhat guilty, had only brought work.

That particular morning, however, I just could not go down to have my *caffè latte* with a social work text, so I picked up Boff's (1985) *Church: Charism and Power.* As I read, I recall thinking: "social workers don't often write like this anymore"–even though I knew that, in Boff's passionate defense of the poor and oppressed, and in his plea to rethink the role of an institution which had become much too concerned with its own power and status, many social workers would feel, as I did, an instant and profound recognition of the ideals that brought us to social work in the first place.

I will not call that moment an epiphany–the notion is too weighty for the light-hearted mood that came with skipping school. But it did bring home to me how timid, as a whole, the social work profession was in standing up for–in caring about, one could even say–the interests of the poor, the marginalized, and the disempowered. And it pushed me to look more closely at what I believed social work to be about, and to translate this more emphatically in my writing, my research and my teaching.

[Haworth co-indexing entry note]: "A Rewarding Group Worker's Journey." Breton, Margot. Co-published simultaneously in *Social Work with Groups* (The Haworth Social Work Practice Press, an imprint of The Haworth Press. Inc.) Vol. 25, No. 1/2, 2002. pp. 23-29: and: *Stories Celebrating Group Work: It's Not Always Easy to Sit on Your Mouth* (ed: Roselle Kurland, and Andrew Malekoff) The Haworth Social Work Practice Press, an imprint of The Haworth Press, Inc.. 2002, pp. 23-29. Single or multiple copies of this article are available for a fee from The Haworth Document Delivery Service [1-800-HAWORTH, 9:00 a.m. - 5:00 p.m. (EST). E-mail address: getinfo@haworthpressinc.com].

23

Not that I had forgotten the ideals that had brought me to social work. The profession, however, was immersed in exploring the plethora of individual and group therapies, and even those who rejected a narrow clinical approach concentrated part of their attention on arguing against it instead of squarely focusing on developing approaches that would lead to both personal *and* social change. (This is the phenomenon sociologists refer to when they point out that, for example, a professed non-nationalist who lives in a nationalist milieu tends to be more nationalist than a professed nationalist who lives in a non-nationalist milieu.)

I could say that I was primed both by my teaching and my work in the community to take up the challenge presented by Boff and liberation theology. During the 1980 academic year, I had taught (as usual) a group work course, insisting that the students make connections between theory and their practicum. After the first class, a student came up to me and explained that she would have to drop out as she doubted she could apply what she would be learning in the classroom in the groups she was working with. I asked her to tell me more about these groups. Well, they were hardly groups to begin with, said she, as their composition tended to change every time they met–"they" being isolated, transient and homeless women residing in one of the larger shelters in Toronto. What the student, who was doing her practicum at St. Christopher House, a neighborhood settlement, was accomplishing with those (granted very open) groups fascinated me, and I persuaded her that she would be able to apply the group work stuff I was teaching. (I also had a soft spot for St. Christ., where I had worked one summer as a day camp counselor before going on to McGill University to get my MSW.)

At the end of the school year, she, her practicum instructor and I met and elaborated a plan for a day-time drop-in for homeless women. An Advisory Board was formed and chose to locate the drop-in in a large, bright room on the ground floor of a community center. This non-stigmatized physical and social environment was very important to the competence-promoting framework we wanted for the drop-in, and I put a lot of thought in developing that framework (1984). Some time later, the Board gathered at St. Christ. House over tea–served, I remember, from a lovely china teapot (those were the days!)–to find a name for the drop-in. After much tea, we came up with *Sistering*, a moniker reflecting the conviction that the women could nurture and learn from each other. I note with a touch of pride that *Sistering* has just celebrated its 20th anniversary and is still going strong.

The book on promoting competence edited by Anthony Maluccio (1981) also influenced my work with *Sistering*, as well as my teaching and writing. Experience as a practicum instructor in the Children's Aid Society of Metropolitan Toronto, a child protection agency, had already convinced me that both students and service users were more likely to get through the tense and difficult situations they faced and learn from them if they thought of themselves–and others thought of them–as having at least the potential competence to do so. The notion of "ecological competence," however, was a breakthrough for me, and I was excited by the possibilities it opened for new ways of thinking about and practicing social work. It transformed my conviction that people can change if others believe in them into a component of a model capable of explaining the presence or absence of competence. With competence seen as resulting from the interaction between an individual's capacities and skills, motivational aspects *and* environment, the "burden" of competence no longer rests solely with the individual. (I had always detested the "blame the victim" aspect of many practice approaches, and it was great to find a model that eliminated both the "blame" and the "victim"!)

My reflections on competence building, along with my close association with *Sistering* and my work as a consultant to practitioners involved with a group of mothers who had neglected or abused (or were at risk of abusing) their children, led me to review the group work literature on the so-called "hard-to-reach" in order to understand their behaviors and develop more effective approaches (Breton, 1985). Based on this research, I posited that these behaviors were purposeful and related to what people learn from past experiences, and concluded that potential users of social work services will be more easily reached and actual users more effectively engaged if their motives–avoiding failure, averting risk and maintaining control–were acknowledged and utilized, and if their strengths were not underestimated. The practice principles I derived were explicitly linked to the provision of opportunities for empowerment. I have to admit I was especially pleased that this model of the behaviors of the "hard-to-reach" which holds the behaviors as rational and situates them in a social learning context, allowed for a different way of looking at what is so often identified as the "resistance" of the "unmotivated"–notions common in social work, and which I have always found profoundly inadequate.

I was lucky to be on a research leave when I was invited to give an opening plenary at the 1989 Group Work Symposium in Montreal, the theme of which was learning from group work traditions. I had the time to examine what three major historical influences on group work–the settlement, the progressive education, and the recreation movements–could teach contemporary group workers (1990). Dipping into the past was a real treat, and I feel terribly sad that many social work curricula no longer include courses on the history of the profession. It was inspiring to see how these movements clearly teach us to look beyond problems and weaknesses, to look at the whole person and not only at the hurt or fragile part of a person, to look at the enormous potential of people to learn throughout life, and at the immense resources a community can offer when the full strength of organized groups is brought to bear on the challenges it and its residents face.

The group work tradition offers an optimistic–not an unrealistic–perception of the world. I was reminded of, and impressed by, the radical way it affirms that challenges can be met and problems solved, but not through following narrow and prescribed paths, not by concentrating on pathology, not by neglecting the transforming power of action and creativity, and especially not in social isolation.

At the Montreal Symposium, I met a group of French social workers who attended a workshop I gave on competence-oriented practice. They were enthused by the approach, and when I went to France the following year, I lectured at various universities and gave workshops in a number of agencies. I thus acquired a sense of how social work can be practiced in a society where socialism and social/collective action are a normal part of life (and are also intensely and widely debated). The concept of partnerships–especially between state and individual or corporate citizens–was a frequent subject of discussion, and I began to see more clearly its relationship and significance to social change and to empowerment.

Joining with others to deal with issues, solve problems, enrich one's social and affective life, have fun, pursue common interests, etc., lies at the heart of group work and of the concept of mutual-aid. It seemed to me that the notion of partnerships added an important dimension to joining, for if there are issues or tasks better attended to by affiliating with a small group than by going it alone, there are aspects of these issues or tasks and there are other issues or tasks better attended to by groups joining forces with other groups, and with other partners, than by a single group going it alone. This led me to think about mutual-aid as involving not only intra-group solidarity and its healing power, but inter and extra-group solidarity and its liberating power, and to argue that to the all-in-the-same-boat dynamic of mutual-aid should be added an all-on-the-same-sea dynamic.

The idea that group work is more than working within a small group is not a new one, but it began to take on a different meaning for me. Along with many other social workers, I was increasingly aware of the political dimension of the work inside and outside of the group. That is why I was so strongly attracted to the empowerment paradigm, recognizing it as one built on the essential unity of the personal and the political/social. Paulo Freire's (1970) views of conscientization (that consciousness-raising which leads only to interior awareness and leaves the outside world untouched is nothing but verbiage), and of praxis (his insistence that action without reflection and reflection without action are unjustifiable), as well as his notion of education as the practice of freedom influenced me profoundly and helped me to understand the meaning and sort out the components of an empowerment-oriented practice (1994a), and to explore the relationship between competence-promotion and empowerment (1994b). I later wrote a paper with my husband which looked at the function of empowerment-oriented groups in democracies (1997). Making use of a fairly elaborate model of democracy, we were able to show that empowerment through groups is essential for the successful (optimal) working of democratic systems. That, in my eyes, further confirmed that the notion of empowerment was a robust one.

These various reflections led me to examine more carefully the role of communities as essential support networks. (Previously, in an effort to model group practice with marginalized populations, I had identified work at the community level as an indispensable element of such practice.) I therefore jumped at the chance offered by the 1998 Miami Symposium, the theme of which was resiliency, to study the community, psychology and community social work practice literature in order to explore the links between the resilience of people and that of neighborhoods. I remember how captivated I was when first hearing of the theme. I was sitting with Toby Berman-Rossi and Tim Kelly in Toby's living room, munching on nuts and raisins, as they expounded on the topic.

I immediately thought how fascinating it would be to look at the resilience of neighborhoods. I reckoned that it is only rational to expect that people will be more liable to bounce back from adversity if their neighborhood–the space that surrounds them and has the potential to either support them or drag them down–is provided with the tools or opportunities to bounce back when *it* is struck by calamity. And so I set out to identify those properties of a neighborhood that make it resilient and capable of sustaining the resilience of its residents (2001).

I wanted to continue examining the role of communities, and accepted to write a paper on the development of Canadian community practice. This gave me the opportunity to research what distinguished this practice from American community organization, which I did with the help of my friend and colleague, Ben Zion Shapiro. I discovered that the Canadian community practice tradition insisted less on the role of coordinator of resources than on that of facilitator and provider of information and services. The Canadian approaches were, on the whole, more participatory and more collectivist, which is understandable given that Canada had had for many years an active socialist political party at all levels of government and that its culture, contrary to American culture, never embraced a strong ideology of individualism. Nonetheless, it struck me that early Canadian community practitioners were operating from a rather paternalistic and therefore controlling stance, for even though they consulted with individuals and groups in the community, they still held a great deal of power. An empowerment approach would have made a difference!

Recognizing social policies as essential instruments of social change, I am intrigued and challenged by the question of how social workers can get groups and communities more involved in policy-making–in becoming informed about and participating in the policy decision-making process. Exploring the connections between social action, social change, social policy and social justice has become more and more important to me, for social injustices cannot be dealt with in any significant way without dealing with the social policies that create or exacerbate them. A passion for justice has been part of my personal make-up as far as I can remember–my mother's unfailing British sense of fair play and my father's profound and rock solid liberalism surely account for this. Moreover, I believe that working towards social change requires social action, which is why using the potential for social action that exists in all groups (as I have argued, 1995), becomes a responsibility for group workers who want to engage in the struggle for social justice.

I have now come to better appreciate the importance, for social workers and the groups they work with, of squarely addressing policy issues and participating in policy change as part of that struggle (forthcoming). I guess I have overcome a latent sense of inadequate preparedness to "think policy" as this was not, in my eyes, within my area of expertise. I, who have so often raved and ranted against social workers' propensity to think in either/or terms–either engage in social change or in individual change efforts–have been somewhat slow in realizing that there is no need to think of policy work as disconnected from community work or group work. All of it is social work, all of it part and parcel of social work's functions. So, to all the readers of *Social Work with Groups*, may I say that it is never too late to learn!

And, I should add, it is never too soon to take a break from one's routine, and go and sip a *latte* somewhere nice with a good (non-social work) book . . .

REFERENCES

Boff, L. (1985). *Church: Charism and Power*. New York: Crossroad.

Breton, M. (1984). "A Drop-In for Transient Women: Promoting Competence Through the Environment," *Social Work*, 29 (6), 542-546.

Breton, M. (1985). "Reaching and Engaging People: Issues and Practice Principles," *Social Work with Groups*, 8 (3), 7-21.

Breton, M. (1989). "Liberation Theology, Group Work, and the Right of the Poor and Oppressed to Participate in the Life of the Community," *Social Work with Groups*, 12 (3).

Breton, M. (1990). "Learning from Social Group Work Traditions," *Social Work with Groups*, 13 (3), 21-34.

Breton, M. (1994a). "On the Meaning of Empowerment and Empowerment-Oriented Practice," *Social Work with Groups*, 17 (3), 23-37.

Breton, M. (1994b). "Relating Competence-Promotion and Empowerment," *Journal of Progressive Human Services*, 5 (1), 27-44.

Breton, M. (1995). "The Potential for Social Action in Groups," *Social Work with Groups*, 18 (2/3), 5-13.

Breton, M. (2001). "Neighborhood Resiliency," *Journal of Community Practice*, 9 (1), 21-36.

Breton, M. (forthcoming). "Empowerment Practice in Canada and the United States: Restoring Policy Issues at the Center of Social Work," *Journal of Social Policy*.

Breton, M. (with A. Breton) (1997). "Democracy and Empowerment," in A. Breton, G. Galeotti, P. Salmon and R. Wintrobe eds., *Understanding Democracy: Economic and Political Perspectives*, (New York: Cambridge University Press), 176-195.

Freire, P. (1968). *Pedagogy of the Oppressed*. New York: Herder and Herder.

Maluccio, A. N. (Ed.) (1981). *Promoting Competence in Clients: A New/Old Approach to Social Work Practice*. New York: Free Press.

The Magic of Mutual Aid

Dominique Moyse Steinberg

> The notes are like us. They don't mean
> much when alone but all when together.
> –Blanche Honegger Moyse

Mutual aid has always been the heart of my professional work. And why not? It has been a powerful force throughout my life, long before I ever heard the term or thought about social work as a career. The last child of a large and musical family that emigrated to this country from Europe after World War II, I grew up in an environment in which it was a norm for people to help one another in common cause. In fact, long before I arrived on the scene mutual aid was essential to my family in order to survive World War II in the middle of Occupied France; and throughout my childhood I heard stories from parents, grandparents, siblings, and extended family about getting by, getting through, and getting on. And while I did not realize it then, what strikes me with great clarity now as I reflect on my professional-practice value system is that inherent in all those survival stories was the need for and reliance on some form and degree of mutual aid.

Surviving as new immigrants in this country also required mutual aid. With a core group of nine, individual strengths were routinely identified, harnessed, and then used for personal and common good. There was a large old house to share, repair, and maintain; gardens to cultivate; a huge back yard to be mowed; fruit trees to be picked; jars and cans to be prepared for wintertime in Vermont; and homemade bread to

[Haworth co-indexing entry note]: "The Magic of Mutual Aid." Steinberg, Dominique Moyse. Co-published simultaneously in *Social Work with Groups* (The Haworth Social Work Practice Press, an imprint of The Haworth Press, Inc.) Vol. 25, No. 1/2, 2002, pp. 31-38; and: *Stories Celebrating Group Work: It's Not Always Easy to Sit on Your Mouth* (ed: Roselle Kurland, and Andrew Malekoff) The Haworth Social Work Practice Press, an imprint of The Haworth Press, Inc., 2002, pp. 31-38. Single or multiple copies of this article are available for a fee from The Haworth Document Delivery Service [1-800-HAWORTH, 9:00 a.m. - 5:00 p.m. (EST). E-mail address: getinfo@haworthpressinc.com].

31

be baked every other day or so. In other words, mutual aid was essential to keeping the family alive and returning it to health. My grandparents, who lived in an upstairs apartment, frequently ate with us, and sometimes we ate upstairs with them. No matter which, however, it seemed like more often than not a friend or colleague or music student joined us at the table so that often the core group of nine became ten, eleven, twelve, and even more at many dinner times. Naturally, in good old-fashioned European tradition, the men tended to drift into an aperitif while the women worked, but even those moments were usually connected by friendly inter-group chatter on subjects of common interest that provided continuing intellectual food for thought over the meal.

Between meals, various musical configurations could be heard in almost every room: my father and grandfather at flute, my mother at violin, my brothers at flute or piano, my sister at piano, and me at violin and piano. Granted, much of this practice time was devoted to individual study, but it was almost always in preparation for some kind of future group process beginning with collective rehearsals and culminating in a local performance or The Moyse Trio on European tour or a chamber ensemble with friends at Marlboro Music School and Festival or some other musical production, such as public-school concerts for children. In other words, it was in preparation for some kind of activity that required both individual and collective contribution and collaboration to succeed.

For example, not only does a Beethoven string quartet need four musicians, it needs collective investment. It needs each player to develop an understanding of and appreciation of his or her role in and contribution to both process (playing certain notes and understanding their relationship to the notes of others) and result (producing the intended music). It needs each player to develop an understanding and appreciation of how all of their roles, together in spiritual and physical synchronicity, synergy, and complementarily contribute to create a work of art, a whole that is greater than the sum of its individual parts. It needs each player to understand and appreciate that without one another's unique contributions neither their individual or collective goals could be achieved. Each person's quality of investment matters a great deal to the honor and integrity of the final artistic production; but no production at all could take place without the participation of each player, whether first or second violin, whether sitting or standing, whether at the front of the group or back. The presence, personal contribution, and mutual appreciation of each is necessary and integral to success.

Getting the members of this large household group where they needed to be when they needed also required mutual aid. Theoretically, there were two cars available, but one car was usually out of commission because my grandfather was far more interested in practicing his flute than "fiddling" with his car! Thus, who needed to be where and when and how to make it happen often took discussion, prioritizing, collaboration, and cooperation. And until the first television was purchased in the mid 1960s, evenings were for gathering in the living room to listen to music (considered to be a *non*verbal activity for "serious" musicians!) and to engage in mutual aid in order to reflect upon and review the nature and quality of the music, performance, and recording.

Most summers were spent at Marlboro, where mutual aid was also the norm. The Marlboro Music School and Festival was the very first summer music festival in this country to be devoted to the practice and performance of chamber music. Co-founded by my parents, violinist Blanche Honegger Moyse and flutist Louis Moyse, along with my grandfather, flutist Marcel Moyse, pianist Rudolf Serkin, and violinist Adolph Busch, this group composed of long-time family, friends, and colleagues developed an ongoing musical community in which groupness and mutual aid predominated. Music was usually practiced and performed in groups. Meals were eaten at long tables of eight or ten, after which one group would clean up the dining hall, another would set up the small stage for a concert by whichever ensemble felt prepared or perhaps set up a portable screen and projector for a Charlie Chaplin film. And at the end of the evening, everyone would help clean up and clear up again in anticipation of the next day of community life filled with a sense of personal and interpersonal need, respect, contribution, and fulfillment.

A few months ago, I offered to help my mother write a short publicity piece on how she became so attached to the man and work of Johann Sebastian Bach. Her first real memory, she said, was of being touched to tears by the Saint Matthew Passion at the age of eight and of then being able to hum much of it by heart long after the concert was over. Little did she realize then, she sighed, where that early experience would eventually lead her professional interest. As she said that, however, I understood with something akin to epiphany, the strength of the threads that connect my early personal experiences of groupness to my professional interest in mutual aid–experiences that were both positive and negative.

Positive experiences were always those that reflected some form of mutual aid: helping others and being helped in a climate of good will, mutual respect, mutual reward, common ground, and collaboration;

recognition of needs and appreciation of strengths; and personal and interpersonal efforts toward a common purpose. Negative experiences, on the other hand, were always those where competition was promoted at the expense of collaboration, fear and insecurity ruled the climate, and differences were either devalued or outrightly derided. As I moved through grade school and high school, feeling safe in some groups and unsafe in others, there were more than just a few in which exclusion rather than inclusion was the dominant value; in which individual personality and accomplishment were valued over interpersonal connections, and in which conformity was demanded–an ongoing observation that eventually provided a dramatic contrast to the earlier experiences of safe and loving groups and that led me, like many other people, to become "group shy."

It was to my own surprise, therefore, when I checked off the "group work major" option with no hesitation on my application to Hunter College School of Social Work many years later and to my even greater mortification that I found myself tongue-tied when asked to talk in my first class about that choice. With what seemed to me like no real experience in group work, I felt incapable of articulating a rationale and mumbled something about having worked for some time in a senior center where many elderly came for lunch, that I had noticed that they always squabbled over seats and food, and that I wanted to gain some skills for helping to bring a sense of order to such a chaotic and "disorganized mess." Immediately embarrassed at such an inept response, I then became preoccupied with trying to understand my own choice of group work over the other options. Now, more than 20 years later, I think how strange to have been so inarticulate about a professional choice with which I now feel in complete harmony and how self-evident it is that promoting mutual aid should have become a professional *cause celebre.*

Some years later, I found myself arguing passionately for a dissertation study on the relationship between social work education and mutual aid; and at one point in the conversation it was suggested that there is more to group work than mutual aid . . . yes? Very conscious of my student status, I responded, "Oh, of course," although in fact, I wasn't at all sure I agreed. Of course context of practice is important, I thought to myself afterward, but why? Of course planning is important. Of course group purpose is important. Of course content is important. Of course nature of membership is important. Of course size of group is important. Of course approach to practice is important. Of course many, many variables are important in forming and working with groups. But why? Why, ultimately, are they important? Why should we think about them?

Spurred by these questions, I continued to explore my own feelings about and attitude toward the place, role, and meaning of mutual aid in social work with groups; and as I did so, I became increasingly convinced that every single theoretical finger points to mutual aid as the *raison d'etre* of this professional method. The belief that people can help one another get by, get through, and get on and that doing so has both intrinsic and extrinsic reward rings loud and clear throughout the group work literature; and today, I am convinced that it is to the end of creating such opportunities that context of practice and purpose is considered, that planning is carried out, that content is selected, that individual membership and overall group characteristics are determined, and that approach to practice is important.

As many opportunities as exist for mutual aid there are opportunities to actually do so. And therein lies the beauty of it. Mutual aid is both an ideal and a reality. As a social ideal, it states that possibilities for helping others and being helped are limitless; as a social *work* ideal, it states that possibilities for catalyzing such a process are limited only by lack of understanding or imagination (Steinberg, 1997). That people should live in ways that promote mutual regard, respect, understanding, and appreciation is an ideal that not only all of the great religions ask for, but that is understood to further the civilization of all life form (Kropokin, 1908). As a reality, mutual aid is a process in which we can engage at many levels and at all times and can be catalyzed if we understand what it means to be truly and profoundly helpful. And it is just this understanding and the conscious, consistent, and even relentless attempt to give real-world meaning to the theoretical value of mutual aid that is the hallmark of social work with groups.

Mutual aid comes in a variety of packages. It can be as dramatic as a heated and passionate debate of differences between two nations in which respective needs, desires, and goals are expressed and explored, as long as they do so in a climate of good will and common desire for better insight, understanding, and empathy. Or it can be as subtle as a nod of recognition from a fellow group member at just the "right" moment.

Furthermore, the right to be helped is a fundamental and universal one, and the privilege and responsibility of helping is not reserved to just the professional. As anyone who loves social work well knows, helping others has great intrinsic reward. We are certainly not in social work for money or other external rewards, such as high social status.

We are in it because helping others is something that gives our own lives meaning. It gives us a reason to be. It gives us a reason to do. It strengthens our personal lives and enriches our interpersonal lives. Why, then, would we not inherently, automatically, and always wish to pass on such opportunities to those people we call clients? Have we come to confuse strength with power? Is it really possible that helping to create venues through which people identify and exchange strengths for personal and interpersonal good could ever weaken the strength of the catalyst? Or have we lost sight of some important connections?

Connections, including those between people, between theory and practice, between needs and group purpose, between worker and members, and even the psyche of needing help and the psyche of being helpful, have always been integral to social work with groups. *Vertical* connections which link generation after generation of group workers, are important because they tie present efforts to both past and future insights. They prevent us from constantly reinventing professional wheels. They force us to anchor our practice with groups in the success (and failures) of those who came before and by "listening up" to these connections, we help to keep our practice true to such fundamental social work values as the right to respect, self determination, and political voice. That is, we keep our group work practice within the realm of *social* work. Some vertical connections are dramatic, like those that tie the purpose of today's fifth-grade after-school club to the intent of professional giants like Grace Coyle. Some are less dramatic, like those that tie the purpose of each group meeting to the other. Whichever the case, however, they mandate us to recognize both the right and capacity of people to have a say over their own affairs, which is but one of many ways to engage in mutual aid.

Horizontal connections, which provide linkages in the here and now, are also important because they are the "stuff" of group work. By connecting the needs we see with possibilities for group purpose, we develop vision. By connecting intent with professional action, we translate vision into work. By helping members connect with one another on a variety of levels, we help them identify common ground and through that common ground, in what ways they can help themselves and one another. And by catalyzing such a process, we remain connected to the *raison d'etre* of social work with groups.

Catalyzing mutual aid is the heart and soul of *social work* practice with groups. Based on the professional belief that whatever its nature, help is best given and taken when a relationship exists, mutual-aid practice does just that: It seeks to establish a relationship not only between the worker and group members in the name of professional help but among members as well in the name of creating exponential sources of help. Based on the professional belief that people have an inherent right to contribute to the shape of their own destinies, mutual-aid practice encourages group autonomy and even helps members to stretch their capacity to do so, both inside and outside the group. And based on the professional assumption that all people have strengths that can be identified and used for personal, interpersonal, and collective good, mutual-aid practice promotes the kind of interaction that best reaches for and harnesses those strengths.

Some years ago, I proposed a parenting group to the director of a group home for pregnant teenage girls where I was working as an intern. To me, the setting was a natural one for group work but I never saw any groups whatsoever except for staff meetings! "Oh," she responded. "We've tried groups here, but they've never worked out." Not prepared to give up so easily, I continued to argue my case and was eventually given permission to go ahead. I diligently planned, researched, and prioritized potential needs, distributed outreach materials, and extended personal invitations as well. Six girls came to the first meeting and, much to the amazement of the agency, the group met once a week for several weeks. I was not amazed, however. I knew that the chance to talk with others in the same boat in a climate of safety would be irresistible. I knew that the chance to share both the pain and wisdom that had been accumulated through their short but poignant life experiences would be irresistible. I knew that the chance to be recognized and respected as contributors to the helping process would be irresistible. In other words, I knew it would be magic.

It is always magical to discover the things about ourselves that are seen as truly helpful by others and to discover the things about others that are truly helpful to us. Was it always simple to catalyze mutual aid in this group? No. It was not always easy to help them move beyond the superficial. It was not always easy to help them listen. It was not always easy to help them explore their differences. And it was not always easy to help them see one another as sources of help. But the connection of my vision with their needs and desires kept the spirit of mutual aid alive, even when its reality as process became a bit wobbly; and the connection of my belief in strength-centered practice with their desire for understanding, respect, and appreciation kept that spirit moving toward an ever more stable reality.

Broadly speaking, it can be said that a major social work mandate is to help people exercise their voices, and catalyzing mutual aid does precisely that. When peers exchange ideas, feelings, attitudes, and personal stories in an attempt to help one another think things through, not only do they provide opportunities to identify those voices that have served them well in the past but they create opportunities to learn new voices as well. The process requires a blend of art, skill, and hard work on the part of everyone involved to help make it happen; but when it does, new worlds open up, like magic.

Conflict and competition rage throughout the world today, and we need the magic of mutual aid more than ever. History tells us repeatedly that behind every advance of civilization there is some form of mutual aid (even if we need to dig deeply to find it)–that in the long run, mutuality (whether emotional, intellectual, or material) will always advance the common good (Kropotkin, 1908; Wilson, 1979) because it seeks inclusion, not exclusion; because it is based in faith, not fear; and because it keeps us honest. In the same spirit as George Bernard Shaw, who was once heard to say, "Christianity's a good idea. Too bad no one's ever tried it!" let us say, "Mutual aid's a good idea. Let's do it!"

REFERENCES

Kropotkin, Peter. (1908). *Mutual Aid: A Factor of Evolution*. London, England: William Heinemann.

Steinberg, Dominique Moyse. (1997). *The Mutual-Aid Approach to Working with Groups*, Northvale, NJ: Jason Aronson Inc.

Wilson, Edward O. (1979). *On Human Nature*. Cambridge, Massachusetts: Harvard University Press.

I Hate Conflict, But . . .

Helen Northen

I hate conflict. I grew up in a family that abhorred conflict. My parents were immigrants from Sweden, a country that prided itself on almost two centuries of freedom from war and on the peace efforts it initiated around the world. As a result of his studies and visits, Donald Connery wrote in *The Scandinavians* that he marveled at the Swedish society which was able to "retain its idealism and good sense in a world scarred by brutality" and "The Scandinavians for all their individual characteristics, have similar institutions as well as a common concern for human rights and a common optimism that solutions can be found for even the most vexing of human problems." Conflict is one of these problems.

My family's immigrant status was the source of some prejudice against us, owing to my parents' strange accents. We all wanted to be accepted as Americans: My parents became citizens at the earliest possible time. Our values included fairness, acceptance of differences among nationalities, loyalty to America, cooperation with others, non-violence and peace. These values, however, could not prevent conflict in our daily lives. Naturally, there were sibling rivalries between the five children and with parents, which were usually around who was to get most of the scarce resources or who was most loved and competent. But such conflicts did not end with bodily hurt or psychological abuse. Lucky me! In school and in the neighborhood, too, there were frequent emotionally-laden arguments and fights which I tried to avoid or simply leave.

[Haworth co-indexing entry note]: "I Hate Conflict, But . . ." Northen. Helen. Co-published simultaneously in *Social Work with Groups* (The Haworth Social Work Practice Press. an imprint of The Haworth Press, Inc.) Vol. 25, No. 1/2, 2002. pp. 39-44; and: *Stories Celebrating Group Work: It's Not Always Easy to Sit on Your Mouth* (ed: Roselle Kurland, and Andrew Malekoff) The Haworth Social Work Practice Press, an imprint of The Haworth Press, Inc., 2002, pp. 39-44. Single or multiple copies of this article are available for a fee from The Haworth Document Delivery Service [1-800-HAWORTH, 9:00 a.m. - 5:00 p.m. (EST). E-mail address: getinfo@haworthpressinc.com].

39

When I stayed with the group, I tried to say what I thought might cool things down and bring about peace, seldom effective.

When I became a leader of groups, first as a volunteer and later as a staff member of the Camp Fire Girls, I became increasingly aware of arguments among members. I also became aware of some of the problems that affected the members' group participation and the group's development. I read whatever I could find to guide me in my efforts to become a good leader. I still remember vividly one meeting of a group of adolescent girls. Angie was accused by the treasurer of stealing some of the group's money. She denied it, said, "You're wrong: It's your mistake." The treasurer screamed that it was not her mistake and that Angie was the last one to handle the money. Angie again denied it. Sides were taken, with name calling and threats to quit the club. Ginny ran out, yelling that she did not want to be in the group any longer. Ramona said, "Good riddance." I was paralyzed, but finally got up enough courage to urge the group to calm down. One member announced, "That's the end of the meeting." All of the girls quickly left the room.

My early efforts to deal with conflict in groups tended to be to talk to participants in the conflict separately, try to change the activity or subject, beg the members to stop what they were doing, or try to say something to soothe the anger and fear. These interventions sometimes suppressed the conflict but, of course, did not solve the problems. Ability to engage the members in defining the issue and using the problem solving process in creative ways came later as did the use of confrontation, accompanied with understanding and empathy. Gradually, I have learned that conflict can be constructive *if* it is resolved in ways that are helpful to all the members.

My increasing experience with conflicts in interpersonal relationships among volunteer leaders as well as girls, different in each situation, was a major influence on my decision to enter a School of Social Work. I thought that social work would be the profession in which I could learn how to help people develop positive relationships and prevent interpersonal conflicts that would result in child abuse, loss of friendships, marital separation and divorce, assault and even murder and war. I understood conflict to mean physical or verbal fighting between two or more people, with the intent to hurt or antagonize the opposition. That fits in with definitions in dictionaries: "to clash," "to fight," "to do battle," or "a quarrel or controversy." However defined, it was to be avoided.

In our work with groups, we need to know that the members attempt to get rid of conflict in several ways. According to Gertrude Wilson and

Gladys Ryland, they are: (1) elimination, that is forcing the withdrawal of the opposing person or subgroup; (2) subjugation or domination, including majority rule, in which the strongest members influence others to accept their point of view; (3) compromise in which each party gives up something in order to safeguard the common areas of interest; and (4) integration or consensus, through which a group reaches a solution that is both satisfying to each member and more creative and productive than any contending position. In group work, we use the problem solving process in attempting to help members reach the latter solution. I hate conflict when efforts to resolve it result in elimination or subjugation, but I love it when the result is integration.

Conflict in practice with groups is usually defined simply as disagreement between two or more participants, including that between workers and members. In that sense, I do not hate conflict. Indeed, recognition of disagreements may be the essence of positive relationships and group life. Acceptance of difference is a basic value of social work. People have a right to express their feelings, ideas, and opinions about happy experiences or devastating ones, as well as problems and their solutions. Verbal communication about the differences is stimulating, providing opportunity for members to learn from each other and assess their own views in relation to those of others.

As differences are discussed, alternative ideas about the issues involved are expressed and solutions offered. As this happen, the agreement and disagreements among the members become clarified: The problem solving process is at work. When members feel satisfied with their efforts to resolve the problem, the relationships among them are strengthened because differences have been accepted, rather than remaining covertly below the surface. For such positive outcomes to occur, there needs to be a social environment in which disagreement is acceptable, even valued. The successful resolution of conflicts strengthens the consensus within the group and enables members to move toward accomplishment of their goals.

I have found that in many groups resolution of interpersonal conflicts is exceedingly difficult. As members interact, their problems outside the group may interfere with their ability to focus on the issue. When conflict is instigated by fears or unconscious processes, when it threatens self esteem or deals with major values, it will be hard to resolve. As conflict accelerates the degree of commitment to one's own position increases. Distortions of perceptions, negative transference reactions to the worker or other members, denial of facts, or emotional and behavioral contagion tend to magnify and perpetuate conflict. Cohesion is low. Workers need to understand the connection between intrapersonal, interpersonal, and group conflict.

I believe that we have tended not to make sufficient distinctions between functional and dysfunctional or harmful conflict. There is little question that conflict, if resolved without harm to anyone, has potentially positive affects. But, it can also be destructive and dysfunctional. There are groups in which conflict is characterized by expressions of hatred or extreme anger, threats to remove particular members from the group, and physical fights. I still cringe when I observe or read about such behavior that hurts people, physically or psychologically. When conflict remains unresolved, it may accelerate the anxiety and fears of at least some members, adding to their difficulties and resulting in drop-outs from the group. The group itself may disintegrate. When conflict occurs in which one or more members feel rejected, discrimated against, or physically attacked, mutual aid cannot operate. I still hate that. The worker should assess the potential hurt to members, and, if present, intervene with the use of confrontation, accompanied by empathy for each member.

Over the years, it has become clear to me that working in conflict situations requires the use of knowledge about human behavior and development throughout the life cycle, with special emphasis on interpersonal relationships; the dynamics and development of groups with varied structures and composition; types of needs, interests, and problems for which group work is the treatment of choice; the selection and use of interventions; and the impact of the environment on members and the group. In efforts to understand and intervene effectively, social workers use the problem solving process. In doing so, they:

1. Reflect on their own values, emotions and past experiences with conflict in order to reduce biases and fears. That is engaging in self awareness for a particular purpose.
2. Understand the nature and quality of their own relationships with each member and of inter-member relationships, striving to develop mutual acceptance, empathy, and genuineness among members.
3. Accept the fact that conflict at some level is inevitable, created by differences in the values, cultures and experiences of the members, the interaction among members, and the group's connections with the environment.

4. Understand and act on the distinction between disagreement with ideas, interests or opinions and dislike rejection, or contempt of another.
5. Avoid taking sides with one individual or subgroup: That is divisive and prevents the full expression of feelings, experiences, ideas, and opinions.
6. Create a social environment that is supportive in establishing a free flow of messages and that is accepting of diversity.
7. Remember that the group is the primary agent of change: Work to involve the participation of all members in the process of dealing with conflict.
8. Trust the group to recognize and respond to tension and conflict among members and with the worker up to the point when assessment indicates that professional intervention is necessary.
9. Engage the members in exploration of the common values, interests, and concerns that underlie the differences among them and help members to understand and accept them.
10. Use limits to control conflict, with special focus on confrontation, when the interaction among members is physically or psychologically harmful to one or more members.
11. Follow-up on absences and drop-outs: They are often occasioned by disagreements about key values or by feelings of rejection or not really belonging in the group.

The purpose of many groups is the enhancement of positive relationships and resolution of problems in relationships at home, school, work, or in the community. That is group work's primary contribution to social work. Learning how to resolve conflicts through the group experience is expected to carry over to more effective coping with the conflicts that occur outside the group. That is good. I now believe, however, that we must give more attention to preventing destructive conflict so people can experience the support and empathy that accrues from a sense of competence in developing and maintaining healthy and satisfying relationships in their families and other groups, friendships, and organizations.

Efforts to prevent destructive conflict would include, for example, the use of psycho-educational groups for parents and teachers of young children for the purpose of helping them to learn how to relate to children with acceptance and empathy and to understand and deal with the inevitable conflicts as they occur in daily living. It would include the services of many more social workers in schools to identify and provide early help to children and their parents when children have trouble in getting along with their peers and teachers. It would include the provision of opportunities for people of all ages to pursue recreational, educational, and cultural activities through which they can develop interests and skills and discover potential friends with whom they may develop mutually, non-conflicted relationships. It's probably too much to hope for, but would it not be wonderful if our political leaders could learn to accept differences, resolve conflicts through means other than elimination of the adversary and killing people in wars?

I close with one of my favorite quotations from Robert Kennedy's speech, delivered on the last night of his life. He said, "I think that the motive that should guide all of us, that should guide all mankind, is to tame the savageness of man and make gentle the life of the world."

Bell Choir, Somersaults,
and Cucumber Sandwiches:
A Journey in Understanding the Importance
of Positive Group Norms

Emily Wolff Newmann

This October I moved to San Francisco from New York City. On my drive across the country, I visited my grandmother in Madison, Wisconsin. She lives at an assisted living facility. While I was there, we attended their Halloween party, a difficult experience for a group worker. No one was talking to each other at the party. Staff were helping people find places to sit, and bringing them ghost and goblin shaped orange cookies and punch with orange sherbet. I wanted the staff to help the residents get to know each other. Some people were singing along or tapping their hands to the music, others were looking at the floor or at the man dressed as Dracula, who was playing his guitar and singing Christmas carols with Halloween themes. After ten minutes of enduring this, my grandmother said, "This could go on for hours." This was my cue that it was time to go.

When we left the party, it didn't surprise me that other people were ready to go also. I wondered if any of the staff members led activities that were engaging and helped the residents get to know each other. The next day, we went to Bell Choir. On the way there, we passed Dorothy, my grandmother's friend, in the hallway. She was twenty minutes early to Bell Choir practice because she wanted to be sure she didn't miss it.

[Haworth co-indexing entry note]: "Bell Choir, Somersaults, and Cucumber Sandwiches: A Journey in Understanding the Importance of Positive Group Norms." Newmann, Emily Wolff. Co-published simultaneously in *Social Work with Groups* (The Haworth Social Work Practice Press. an imprint of The Haworth Press. Inc.) Vol. 25, No. 1/2, 2002, pp. 45-51; and: *Stories Celebrating Group Work: It's Not Always Easy to Sit on Your Mouth* (ed: Roselle Kurland, and Andrew Malekoff) The Haworth Social Work Practice Press, an imprint of The Haworth Press, Inc., 2002. pp. 45-51. Single or multiple copies of this article are available for a fee from The Haworth Document Delivery Service [1-800-HAWORTH, 9:00 a.m. - 5:00 p.m. (EST). E-mail address: getinfo@haworthpressinc.com].

45

My grandmother loves music. She is 93 years old and can still play show tunes on the piano, all by ear. When we arrived, there were fifteen people already sitting down, many chatting loudly. The wheel chairs and chairs were set up in a circle so everyone could see each other. A tall young man smiled at my grandmother when she walked in and said, "Hi Janet, come on in. Let's make a seat for you over here. I'm so glad you came to bell choir."

Brian had everyone introduce himself/herself before beginning practice. Each person was given a wood block with a bell attached to it. When Brian began, he gave the group a choice of songs to work on that day. Once this was decided he said, "Now I want everyone to make sure you have eye contact with me at all times so you know that when I point to you it will be your turn to play. Everyone will get a chance to play songs today, so if you aren't in the first song hold tight because you will be later on. Okay, deep breath everyone, we need to get ready to play. It's important we sit up straight when we play." People adjusted themselves in their seats and looked attentively at Brian, who was in the middle of the circle.

Brian gestured with his hands and looked at people in the eye, conducting the group members to play a lively Austrian waltz. After they finished, Brian asked the group how they thought it went. One woman, who had been closing her eyes and nodding her head to the rhythm of the waltz, said, "I thought it sounded good." She looked around to see if others agreed with her. A few people nodded and said, "Sounded good." One of the only two men in the group said, "I think it was okay, but we could do better." "Good idea, Mel. How do you think we can make it better?" Brian asked the group. A woman who had not looked at the group the whole time said, "I think maybe we need to make the bells sound clearer, like they do in church." "Thanks for the suggestion, May. Everyone make sure you really make clear sharp strokes with your wrists. Okay, let's try again," Brian said, smiling at the group. One woman was noticeably having a difficult time ringing her bell because her hand was shaking. Brian went over to her and said, "Gloria, try again using both hands to steady the bell. There you go. That was great. Wasn't it?" Brian asked the group. Many people nodded in agreement. A man to Gloria's right leaned over his wheelchair and whispered audibly, "Thata girl." Gloria smiled, seemingly pleased with herself.

I left my grandmother in Bell Choir practice to get back on the road. While it is always hard to leave, I was thrilled to know that my grandmother was part of a group that she enjoyed. Many of the participants had so many disabilities and problems that go along with the territory of growing old, and yet it didn't seem to matter in Bell Choir practice. Brian found a way to include everyone in the choir regardless of their physical and/or mental deficits. From my brief observations, it seemed the group had developed some wonderfully positive group norms, those being: an expectation of equal member participation, an acceptance of each individual's abilities, a sense that every member is important to the group, and lastly, group interaction was encouraged while making music together. It was quite a stark contrast to the Halloween party the day before.

Four years earlier, when I started at the Hunter College School of Social Work in 1997, I don't think I would have observed bell choir practice the way I did a few weeks ago. I probably would have enjoyed it, but I don't think I would have been quite as aware of how the group members were interacting with each other. While I didn't know the term "group norms" before I went to social work school, I now recognize how my experiences in groups throughout my life influenced my belief in positive group norms before I had a language to describe them. Over the past four and a half years, through observing groups and applying Social Group Work principles, combined with my own values, to practice, I have gained a deeper understanding of how important positive group norms are to the success of a group.

We participate in groups since the time we are young. There are so many groups to be part of: girl scouts, little league, book clubs, bridge groups, foot ball teams, debate clubs, office happy hour, band practice, and the list goes on. I remember being ten years old and rushing to get to my gymnastics team practice because I couldn't wait to see everyone. Everyday when I walked into that gym, Manny, my coach, said, "Hey Gumby," (I was flexible) with a big smile, and then I would go warm-up with the girls on the big blue mat. Everyone on the team had nicknames, which celebrated a unique quality about the person. While now I can describe some of the positive group norms of the gymnastics team, then I just knew I liked how I felt when I was there. They were about helping each other out, taking risks, never giving up, being serious about your practice without taking yourself too seriously, and learning from everyone's unique abilities.

There is nothing unusual about these norms; however, it was the way they were developed that made the experience so meaningful and formative. Our coach set the tone of the group. He pushed us to do our best, and in this group culture of determination he taught us to smile and cheer and pat each other on the back as we flipped and turned and fell on our faces, only to get back up again. There were times we would be in tears from frustration or pain, and Manny gave us encouragement with a hug or a smile, or often said, "Give it a rest today. We'll work on that tomorrow. It will come." He treated us with respect. By modeling this for us, we learned how to have respect for ourselves, and one another.

In my first group in Social Work School, I realized I was the one to set the tone. I had led groups before in previous jobs working with young people, however, this time I was more conscious of my role in creating a positive group culture. The group members were 5th and 6th graders in an after-school program. After playing a few icebreakers to help everyone feel more comfortable, my co-leaders and I divided the group into smaller groups of about five people to work on creating group expectations or the "ground rules." Each group was given a piece of large brown paper that was cut out in the shape of a person; it was called a "dough person." They were instructed to write down on the inside of the dough person what they wanted in the group, and on the outside they had to write what they didn't want to happen in the group. Kids were busy with markers writing down short commands. The papers were filled with some of the following words: "Respect each other," "Listen," "Be nice," "Don't say Shut Up!!" "Fun," "Don't tell secrets," "No Fighting," "Make friends," "Participate," "Share," "Say how you feel," "No Dissing," "Be Honest," "Don't laugh at people if they make a mistake."

These suggestions became the fundamentals of the group norms. As the group progressed, they became internalized and second nature to the group. There were times when kids needed reminders of the expectations, and often the members were the ones to do this. Because the members felt safe in the group, the norms of participating, speaking out, working together, trying new things, making decisions together, and treating each other with respect were relatively easy to adjust to.

One day when the group was in middles, the majority of the group was protesting an activity I was leading. It was, "stupid" and "whak" and group all of a sudden was "boring." Some kids were sitting down and refusing to play this cooperative game. "Why do we have to play games you make up?" John asked. The tension was thick. Eyes were rolling all over the place. One girl said, "C'mon let's just do it so we can get to the other stuff. It's not that bad." While I felt like sitting the group down and talking about respect, instead I took a deep breath and asked the group why it was so "boring" and what they wanted to do. After a heated conversation about how the group wanted to play more of the games they knew and liked, we came to a resolution. We had reminded the group that in the past they liked things they had never tried. Melissa, an internal leader suggested, "We should do both." The group voted on how we should work it out. While in the beginning, I felt frustrated with what seemed to me defiance, later I was able to see how internalized norms were actually at work in the messy stage of middles. The group had gotten to a place where they were comfortable enough with each other and us (leaders) to challenge what was going on and make a group decision. Something we had been working on all along!

I soon found out that all groups were not run with positive group norms in mind. My second year placement was at a day treatment center for adults diagnosed with mental illness. The clients spent the majority of their time in groups. In observing groups, I noticed that some group leaders didn't even look at all the members of the group. They gave all their attention to the people who were verbally participating or even monopolizing. This had become the norm. When I asked about it, I would often hear, "X never speaks. I don't even think he knows what is going on." Another thing that surprised me was that when groups were canceled, other group leaders would fill in for each other. Group members were rarely notified ahead of time, or asked what they wanted to do if a facilitator was going to be absent. The latent message was "The group is not important, anyone can run it." This way of treating groups seemed very disrespectful.

I decided I wanted to create a group where people would not only feel welcome, but dignified. A place where people would want to come, relax, and get to know each other in an intimate environment which suggested to those entering that they were valued. Many of the clients who attend the day treatment program reside in assisted living residences. Their lives are often regulated by agency policies, both at the day treatment program and at home. Whom they room with, what time they need to be home, when they eat, what they eat, where they eat are often determined by their housing program. Most people eat two or three meals a day on plastic or paper plates in rooms void of any personal meaning. People file in and file out, for the dining room does not invite lingering conversation. The goal was to create a group that suggested to those attending a sense of dignity, first from the atmosphere and second, from the way in which the group would be facilitated. Thus, the "High Tea" group was born.

The cucumber sandwiches and grapes were laid out on the table next to the mugs. Pat was sitting by the coffee machine vigilantly watching each drop fill up the pot a little bit more. Every so often she would say, "The hot water is ready for tea." Pat had offered to help set up and seemed to be enjoying the responsibility of this task. On the table the candles glowed. Tom took on the role of the helper; he began asking people what they would like to drink and pouring the tea for those who were sitting down. The noise in the room was a combination of Mozart's violin concertos resonating from the CD player, the rustle of people helping themselves to the food and drinks, and the voices of those engaged in conversation.

I noticed that many people seemed somewhat solemn. The discussion in the group that day was about how people were feeling tired and stressed out recently. As Charlie was speaking, Jay had his head down and was hunched over in the corner, almost seeming to be trying to disappear. Jay had come to this group twice, but had never said a word. I looked around the room to see if other people were looking at Jay. A few people were, but nobody said anything to him. Cathy looked concerned. I said, "Jay, you have been quiet, and I am wondering what you are thinking about?" Everyone waited attentively to hear what he had to say. After about a minute of silence, Jay said deliberately and slowly, "I am dealing with the loss of my brother right now." Silence. It seemed people did not know how to respond at first. I made eye contact with Jay from across the room and said, "Death is always really difficult to deal with. No matter if you expect it, you are never quite prepared." "It's really hard. My father died a year ago and I still have a hard time when I think about it," Ann said. Maria said, "My cousin recently died, I have had a lot of people I know die. I have dealt with a lot of loss. It's very difficult." "I lost my father four years ago and I never cried when he died. I still haven't and it still bothers me," Charlie said. Jay listened now with his head up, looking at whomever was speaking. Cathy was sitting next to Jay. She put her hand on his shoulder and said, "Thanks, Jay, for telling us. Let us know what we can do for you." Jay looked at her and said softly, "Thank you, I feel better just talking about it."

Not every group can be a "High Tea" group; however, after a few years of experience I am convinced that dignity needs to be at the heart of building positive group norms. We feel good about ourselves when we are treated with respect and are valued. We crave this. So much of the work of building positive group norms has to do with our values and how we interact with people. We set the group tone. As group leaders, we are setting norms all the time, and yet I don't think we think about it. We are setting norms when we make eye contact with group members as we scan the group, give smiles of encouragement, call people by their names, and acknowledge who is absent and who has returned. It is happening when we facilitate group decision making, normalize feelings, create opportunities for full member participation, set limits, allow people to express all kinds of emotions in and about the group, and by all the other subtle and explicit ways we communicate with group members. It becomes second nature.

Over the past two years, in my work with African-American and Latina teenage girls, I became more aware of how positive group norms are influenced by the blending of the members' and leader's cultural norms, values, and communication styles. I struggled with how much I should encourage the girls to accept my values. For example, I wanted to foster a respectful way of communicating, and yet the girls had their own language and communication style based on their youth culture. When they spoke to each other they often would put each other down; this was their way of joking around and showing affection. In my first girls groups, I used to insist that they did not make fun of each other. During group sessions, there were times when girls would speak to each other as they do outside of group, and then look at me and apologize. I felt uncomfortable with this. So we talked about how it was not always clear to me if they were joking, and how at times it seemed like people got offended. Some girls spoke out about how they didn't like all the "dissing." Just by talking about it and discussing semantics, we built more trust in the group and girls seemed to think more about what they said before making fun of each other. We agreed that the members should be able to speak to each other as they always do, but anyone in the group could say "ouch" if they were offended by something someone said. Figuring out a norm of group communication that was both positive, and did not strip the girls of their cultural language, was something I became more comfortable with over time.

In watching the girls grow over the past two years, I noticed how many of the girls who participated in my first groups started communicating and interacting with each other in more positive ways outside of the group. It was wonderful to see how positive group norms not only influenced a group's interactions, but also became ingrained in the girls' values and behaviors. They are so important!

Now I have begun a new journey. I am sitting at my kitchen table in my San Francisco apartment having my own high tea, thinking of my grandmother in Bell Choir practice. This journey of understanding the importance of positive group norms is completed, but the road to building them is in front of me.

Grizzly Empathy

Mary Bitel

When I was asked last summer to write about empathy, I cheekily thought, "Oh gosh, what could be easier? I *know* empathy when I see it; this is a task I can polish off in a weekend," and promptly put the project out of mind. I went about the summer planning program for my agency while teaching acting to N.Y.U. theater majors, topped off with a trip to Juneau, Alaska in late August. As the summer wore on, I knew there was something I was neglecting. I had that nagging, pit-in-the-stomach kind of feeling that I get when I realize I'm avoiding something *big*. As I sat by a river at salmon spawning time trying to figure out why I was feeling increasingly uncomfortable, I watched a grizzly bear chomping away on his freshly butchered salmon lunch. The tourists were flocking, great hordes of them, happy to have captured a Kodak moment as they snapped away on their cameras in their own feeding frenzy. The poor bear's private moment was exposed to the world in an artificial glare of video camera lights and flashbulbs. I felt absolute empathy for the poor grizzly . . . or so I thought in the moment.

The more I reflected on the plight of the grizzly, however, the more I realized that I couldn't fit my feelings for the bear into my favorite definition of empathy. This definition comes by way of Roselle Kurland and Helen Northen and is attributed by them to an anonymous English writer. They quote the writer as telling us that empathy is the ability "to see with the eyes of another, to hear with the ears of another, and to feel with the heart of another" (2001, p. 68). Empathy is, according to *Webster's Dictionary* an "identification with or vicarious experiencing of

[Haworth co-indexing entry note]: "Grizzly Empathy." Bitel, Mary. Co-published simultaneously in *Social Work with Groups* (The Haworth Social Work Practice Press, an imprint of The Haworth Press, Inc.) Vol 25, No. 1/2, 2002, pp. 53-59, and: *Stories Celebrating Group Work: It's Not Always Easy to Sit on Your Mouth* (ed: Roselle Kurland, and Andrew Malekoff) The Haworth Social Work Practice Press, an imprint of The Haworth Press, Inc., 2002, pp. 53-59. Single or multiple copies of this article are available for a fee from The Haworth Document Delivery Service [1-800-HAWORTH, 9:00 a.m. - 5:00 p.m. (EST). E-mail address: getinfo@haworthpressinc.com].

53

the feelings or thoughts of another." It took me a while, but as I watched the grizzly and the tourists in action and reflected on my first-hand experiences with empathy in social group work practice I realized that what I was really experiencing was good old-fashioned sympathy.

Webster's defines sympathy as an "agreement in feeling, as between persons"–in other words, to respond with feeling to another's situation. Empathy implies a relationship to another that has its connection in lived experience; to take in and be affected by others' feelings and issues because of a personal connection made to one's own experiences. Well, I may be going out on a limb, but I would hazard a guess that the grizzly bear was not terribly concerned with how any of us camera-toting humans were connecting to his experience. And I seriously doubt he needed my full understanding in order to meet his emotional needs. The bear was a lot bigger than any of us, so he had nothing to fear from the reactions of the group. He was simply storing up for the anticipated Alaskan winter. I was merely projecting my own feelings onto those of the grizzly. It was in that moment that I was able to identify the source of the pit-in-the-stomach feeling. I realized that the thing I had been so nonchalant about in June, mainly my assumptions about my understanding of empathy, was coming back to haunt me. The irony is that empathy is so obviously vital to my work and so simple in its definition that it is too elusive to put easily into words. When I tried to define empathy in my work, I felt as though I was trying to grab hold of something as elusive and slippery as the salmon flopping about in front of me.

My Alaskan encounter reminded me that I was on my own journey from sympathetic friend, teacher and administrator to empathic professional. As I share my experiences and knowledge base with staff and students, as I look at the world around me, I am seeing that empathy is at the core of practice. At the same time, empathy has become the subject I find most elusive and difficult to teach. Can one be taught to be an empathic person? I don't believe so. Can one be taught to *use and develop* one's capacity for empathy as a tool in social work practice? Absolutely. A vital piece of that teaching is helping students to make a very clear distinction between two different emotional responses. Most often, I hear my staff and students respond with genuine concern and need to "help" their clients, but are they speaking from a place of empathy or one of sympathy? The two are often easily confused by well-meaning practitioners. While sympathy strikes at our need to fully invest our emotions, it doesn't necessarily imply the work of self-reflection and distance required in empathy to move from subjective experience to the objectivity necessary to assist others toward self-growth.

I returned from my summer odyssey to New York in September of 2001 and to my work as an administrator, field instructor and group worker. The article had yet to be written and putting my thoughts about empathy down on paper seemed just as elusive as ever. I sat one late fall afternoon facilitating a discussion on body image in a group of ten adolescent girls. One member, a 13-year old we'll call Tawna, was describing her recent confrontation with a group of peers over her choice of clothing–not designer label apparel, but an outfit her mother had picked out because there was little money in the family budget to spend on clothing. I listened in, noting the discomfort on several faces in the circle as Tawna shared her story. How many times had each of us made a judgment about someone else based on his or her outer appearance? More to the point, how many of us had been on the receiving end of such judgment?

As I struggled to understand my own feelings and responses to issues being raised in the group, I was increasingly aware of how important it is to allow those feelings in to understand the content and apply it to the group–*in the moment*. My understanding of empathy in this context was based on my own early experiences. Tawna's story hurtled me back twenty-four years to eighth grade, Lowell Junior High School, Livonia, Michigan, the first day of co-ed volleyball. I was shunned by the girls that day and many days after that as too un-cool in my owl-rimmed glasses and lack of late-70s make-up. I was spurned by the boys who preferred teammates who giggled, dropped the ball and wore the "right" gym apparel. I remember my mother offering me words of support and sympathy. Still, she sent me back to gym purgatory the next day in the same outfit.

Flash forward twenty-four years and across half the continent to my stalwart band of girls in East Harlem. I scanned the faces of the members, took a deep breath and remarked, "It sounds like Tawna is having a rough time of it at school. *(Turning to Tawna)* It also sounds like you're saying that people don't really appreciate you for what's underneath the outer layers. I'm wondering if anyone else has had that experience–of not being heard or seen for who you really are." Dead silence; every hand, including my own, raised high. The conversation picked up again after a beat. *(Janet)* "I don't like to go to gym 'cause I get picked on 'cause my sweats smell bad." A few girls laughed and even more nodded their heads in silent support. *(Stacey, turning to Tawna)* "Don't listen to those losers, they're wack." *(Angela)* "Yeah, they don't know the real you like we do. We *know* you're wack but we love you anyway." The girls all joined in the laughter, including Tawna; empathy in action.

What I had wanted as a funny kid with glasses and un-cool gym wear was someone who could understand me for who I was and where I was coming from, not just sympathize with my plight. Sympathy most often has the effect of making the receiver feel "less than" and places the sympathizer in a position of being somehow distanced or "above" the recipient of her kind words or actions. I remember thinking, as that gawky eighth grader, that I didn't want my mother's (or anyone else's) sympathy. I wanted the equality of empathy; I wanted to hear from someone who had walked in my (gym) shoes and knew what it felt like to be there. Tawna received that from her fellow group members. My role as the group leader couldn't have been more clear where empathy is concerned. It was my job to use myself; to take in, to understand, and be sensitive to the experiences and needs of the members and, using the group setting, to assist the group members to gain the ability to practice empathy with each other.

This example is not meant to imply that one must have lived through a similar experience in order to empathize with a client's issues or situation. In the following example, the social worker is a petite, Caucasian woman in her mid-thirties. She sits with a group of inpatient veterans in the recreation room of a veteran's administration hospital in a major urban center. The group is made up of a mix of Caucasian, Latino and African American men, ranging in age from early 20s to late 60s. All group members have been admitted to the hospital for drug related problems. The social group worker has virtually no experience in working with substance abusers and no history of military service.

The group has just completed a simple role-play activity to address difficulties in communicating their individual needs to hospital staff and visiting family members. While the activity had produced lively discussion and much mutual support within the role-play activity to "tell her what you really feel, man!" the group has now fallen silent. The group worker sits with the silence, scanning the faces of the men in the group. Some scowl, others slouch in their seats. More silence, *lots* of it. Finally Leon, a group member, speaks up, "So, what's the point? I mean we're just playin' around in here. What good does it do to practice tellin' them how we *feel?*" More silence. Jim picks up the dialogue, "He's right. No offense, but your acting stuff doesn't really help when it comes to real life." The group worker sits with the feelings for a good 20-count and then speaks, "It can all feel really pointless sometimes, huh?" Jim nods. She continues, "Like, why bother? Anybody else ever feel that?" More nods. She persists, "So why bother?"

She turns to the group member next to her, who had been the most vocal supporter of the last role-play exercise. "Pete, how did it feel when Jim stood up and told his sister how much he needs to see his family?" Pete leans forward in his chair with a beaming smile, "Great, man, really cool." The worker continues, "You seemed pretty involved in what was going on with Jim, like you had some ideas on how you'd want to say something like that if you ever got the chance." Pete shrugs his shoulders and sitting back in his chair remarks, "Yeah, well, he did it good. I mean, sometimes people don't get how hard it is to be here and the regular stuff we need, like just messin' around with the kids." The worker nods and sits quietly with the group. "So I guess even when it feels really pointless, sometimes you've just got to do it anyway if it seems important."

The group moved on to a discussion about the difficulties they face in communicating with family members. The group worker had reached for the connection to the issues and emotions being shared by the group. She had never experienced the humility of being treated like a criminal by family members because of a drug problem. But, she certainly had experienced the feeling of wanting something very much and wondering whether or not hard work and good intentions were enough to achieve her dreams against the heavy odds in front of her. Like the group members, she had more than once found herself wondering what the point was.

Personal experience of being on the receiving end of sympathy has helped me to understand the necessity of empathy in social group work practice and has taught me the value of articulating the difference between the two. Professional experience has taught me that those of us who leap to sympathy as a "quick-fix" connection to a client's issues and dilemmas are short changing the client-worker relationship and throwing a roadblock up in front of real potential for greater self-discovery and growth. The most striking difference between empathy and sympathy is how one uses oneself in relation to others. With empathy, it is not so much how one feels in the moment but how one chooses to relate to others and to her own feelings and then how one uses self-knowledge to get the group moving. To understand this concept as a skill that can be developed and practiced makes the difference between a sympathetic listener and an empathic, active participant in change.

So where am I now in my insights, observations and beliefs about empathy and group work? Well, I guess I'm learning that the ability–or the need–to be empathic in group work practice is not a given. Each practitioner must find the ability to be empathic in her work through her willingness to look at the "stuff" that makes up her own life experiences. Then she has to make the decision about how to use those experiences to help her group to find their own connections to each other. I'm also learning that empathy and sympathy are easily confused in the practice of social group work. This is an essential point for me to be clear about in my practice, as it impacts my ability to be an effective administrator, teacher and group worker.

As an administrator, I am constantly aware on two different levels how my program is progressing. One the one level, I am noting such factors as how many girls are attending programs, how many parents are involved, and how girls are doing overall in building relationships with each other and with staff. On another level, I am constantly taking the "empathy temperature" of my staff and the various groups they facilitate throughout the week. While I am aware that I need to understand the challenges that my staff face in their practice and the various schools of thought and levels of experience they bring to the work, I do believe that being clear about the difference between empathy and sympathy is essential in the practice of good group work. It is vital to be able to understand the difference between empathy and sympathy because it is a skill that I hope for all clients to develop. It is an essential component of the group process.

If you were to ask me where I rate the ability to be empathic as a factor in group work practice, I would tell you that it scores off the charts. I would be lying if I said that I practice strong empathic skills in my work with groups every time out of the gate. Sometimes I don't get it. Sometimes I miss the connection and end up sitting in sympathy. Don't get me wrong, sympathy feels very good initially but always ends up leaving me feeling distanced from the group and without a strong idea of how to proceed. My sympathetic understanding of the situation, often leaves the group members out there feeling the need to be sympathetic to the given situation, but not really taking each other in or using their own connections to similar experiences to help each other move forward.

Here's the positive part about empathy: For every moment of missed connection there are ten-fold moments where the group members make the leap from passive listeners to active providers of mutual aid. They do that through their need to process and share their own experiences and the need to understand each other. And that happens because of the worker's understanding that empathy is only as good as it's passed on to others to share. That's the magic of empathy. That's what connects human beings to each other. Empathy, unlike sympathy, offers hope for change. Now that's something I do know how to write about.

REFERENCE

Northen, H. and Kurland, R. and (2001). *Social work with groups.* (3rd ed.) New York: Columbia University Press.

It Is Not Always Easy
to Sit on Your Mouth

Camille P. Roman

When I first elected to write this piece, I was enticed by the suggestion of the editors to write an article about staying with issues when
working with a group. The request was to make the article "short, personal, and reminiscent in nature." As I thought about the topic, my mind
wandered back to my earliest group experience–my family.

Ah yes, I was soon flooded with warm thoughts of family and home. I
drifted in and out of many places, but the dinner table "discussions"
were particularly vivid. I could once again hear the familiar screams and
yells filling the tiny kitchen where we all squeezed together at night for
our daily supper. I could almost see the occasional flying dish or cup
and hear it smashing against the wall or floor. I remembered how the
tension filled the air. I could hear the old hysterical death threats, the
loud crying and, of course, the violent slamming of doors as one person
or another threatened to leave and "never come back." Ah, the old
sounds of home and hearth!

Growing up in an economically deprived and chaotic family, I struggled with many issues. I was always saddened and confused by how everyone struggled so desperately to be heard and how no-one was ever
listening. Once sitting watching a particularly vitriolic exchange at a
holiday gathering (those holidays were always special), my face apparently betrayed my fear and confusion to an elderly aunt. Tia Mercedes

[Haworth co-indexing entry note]: "It Is Not Always Easy to Sit on Your Mouth." Roman, Camille P.
Co-published simultaneously in *Social Work with Groups* (The Haworth Social Work Practice Press, an imprint of The Haworth Press, Inc.) Vol. 25, No. 1/2, 2002, pp. 61-64; and: *Stories Celebrating Group Work: It's
Not Always Easy to Sit on Your Mouth* (ed: Roselle Kurland, and Andrew Malekoff) The Haworth Social
Work Practice Press, an imprint of The Haworth Press, Inc., 2002, pp. 61-64. Single or multiple copies of this
article are available for a fee from The Haworth Document Delivery Service [1-800-HAWORTH, 9:00 a.m. -
5:00 p.m. (EST). E-mail address: getinfo@haworthpressinc.com]

61

turned to me with her soft face and wise eyes and whispered, "When your tongue is silent only then can you hear." I knew, then, I was not alone in what I saw. This aunt, who was secretly thought to be a witch, knew what I knew, saw what I saw. She was telling me that what I intuitively felt was accurate–something else was going on here, something that was beneath the drama and the noise. All the words that were thrown about and never received didn't really count. The interactions were about something else, and if I didn't get caught in the noise, maybe I could understand and make sense of it. I instinctively knew if I could understand, make sense of the chaos, it would be less frightening and I would not feel so powerless.

Once I came to this realization I felt validated, no longer confused or frightened. No, in fact, I was now on a mission. I was going to figure this out. I was going to find something else, ferret it out and be rid of it! I would be the dragon slayer and save the family and myself along the way. Dragon slayer–social worker–could there be a connection?

Today when I return home for family visits, the familiar smells and sounds still fill the tiny kitchen. Not much has changed. Some members are gone now, some new co-dependent ones have been carefully selected to insure that the family dynamics are kept stable. I still feel and see the "something else," but the major change for me is that I no longer try to, or believe I can, get rid of the dragon. In fact, I see now that the dragon is a necessary part of the group/family, a member if you will.

Upon reflection, it is astounding to me to realize how young I was when I learned to keep an objective and safe distance from the tumult of that early group experience. Perhaps it was my innate survival mechanism that enabled me to be a part of the chaos while keeping a safe distance, or perhaps it was just the witch gene flowing through my blood. Whatever it was, where ever it came from, I have always had a talent for tolerating chaos in groups. Tolerating the chaos and not getting pulled into it enabled me to hear the "something else," the latent content. I was able to see the process of interacting and not get stuck in the content. Being aware of my own feelings enabled me to establish an empathic bond for those struggling to be heard. I learned later in my formal training that feeling and establishing an empathic bond were essential to determine where the group was, but if I became overwhelmed by the feelings I would be rendered helpless as a worker.

The trick for the worker, I learned, is to develop a rhythm. The rhythm, like breathing, involves moving in and moving out of the emotional component of the group. The worker must learn to move in and feel, then move out and process, all the while staying with the feelings.

The difficulty for the worker is to avoid staying too long in the feelings and risking being swallowed up. The demand is to stay long enough to be where the group is and identify the issue. After the identification of the issue is established, it must be processed. That also involves staying with the feelings, but now in a more objective way. After the experience is processed, the worker can help members translate how that experience has had impact on their behavior in the group.

To accomplish all of the above, the worker must learn to "sit on her mouth" (Tia Mercedes again). It is not always easy to sit on your mouth, especially in a chaotic family (oops, I mean group).

For most workers it is a difficult and often frightening thing to tolerate the emotional depth and intensity that a group can engage in. Powerful feelings of rage, sadness, and emptiness can trigger old countertransferential responses in the worker. The worker's old demons can spring forth and prompt various forms of defensive behavior disguised as interventions. The worker may over identify and merge with the group's feelings, consequently feeling safe in the tumult by not challenging it. The worker may ward off his or her own feelings of incompetence and inadequacy by being the expert, and having the answers. The worker may struggle to keep in check a historical need to be loved by not confronting members or by not establishing the role as the professional.

The impulse to protect the self and not allow the group to go where it needs to go in order to do its work, is strong. The worker must stay with the feelings, let them unfold and carry the group wherever it needs to go in order to achieve its goals. The group must be held to the work, no matter how frightening it is for the worker.

When I first began in group work, I could see the process clearly. Latent messages leaped out at me (ah, the old witch gene). Where other workers heard stories from new members about subway problems resulting in chronic late arrivals, I heard fear of engagement related to beginning issues of trust and approach-avoidance. Even more exciting to me was to have my insights validated by my professors and supervisors (my new Tias). With all that encouragement I jumped into action, interpreting what I saw whenever I saw it (the old dragon slayer at work). The subsequent result of my hasty intervention was, of course, to freeze the group's ability to explore. I had not yet learned to "sit on my mouth" (forgive me, Tia).

I have since come to understand that premature intervention short circuits the process of exploration of feelings and that exploration is essential to the group's growth. I also have learned that when a worker intervenes too quickly it is generally the result of that worker's inability to contain some historical defensive impulse. In my case, the impulsive intervention was related to my need to establish order in my chaotic family and thereby to feel safe.

When we too quickly problem solve, reassure, help justify an action, explain away a frightening feeling or in any way intervene without reflection, we are short circuiting the group's work. To properly explore the issues (get to the "something else"), the worker must develop the ability to glide in and out of feelings, helping the group move deeper and deeper. When the worker remains steady, demanding the group to stick to the work, members feel safe, as if being helped to steer through a storm.

With each successful level of exploration, group members become more empowered, ultimately, having consciously experienced, explored and survived their old historical storms. Group members, the worker, and the group as a whole emerge stronger.

AUTHOR NOTE

Special thanks to my Dear Friend Sondra Brandler.

REFERENCES

Billow, R. The Therapist's Anxiety and Resistance to Group Therapy, *International Journal of Group Psychotherapy,* Vol. 51 #2, April 2001.

Brandler, S. and Roman C. (1999) *Group Work Skills and Strategies for Effective Interventions,* 2nd Ed., New York: The Haworth Press, Inc.

Cooper, M., Granucci Lesser, J. (2002) *Clinical Social Work Practice: An Integrated Approach.* Boston: Allyn and Bacon.

Tia Mercedes, Moca, Puerto Rico.

Will the Real Healer Please Take a Bow

Rachel Miller

The program I work in at Hillside Hospital in Glen Oaks, New York is a National Institute of Mental Health research project designed to learn more about the early years of schizophrenia. Although my work is centered in the research division of a large psychiatric hospital, the clinical care I am involved with requires me to work with patients in a continuum of care. This begins with admission and moves through inpatient to day hospital and finally outpatient departments. This means I get to know patients at their most vulnerable, when they come into the hospital for the first time, and continue to work with them as the healing process continues into the community. The groups I facilitate include a day hospital symptom management group which meets five times a week, five outpatient groups which meet once a week each, and a twice monthly family group.

It was about the third year of leading special groups for young people with schizophrenia that I learned to let go of some of the rules of group therapy in order to tap into the strengths of my clients. Maybe I needed the rules to provide me with a sense of control when I was working with an illness that by its nature means a loss of control. Possibly I needed to be fully comfortable with schizophrenia and its many mysteries before I could begin editing the rulebook, but when I started questioning I started at the top.

Over the first two years working in the research study, I often thought of Freud's statement that people with schizophrenia are narcissistic. I was on the watch for that narcissism but did not see it the way I had with

[Haworth co-indexing entry note]: "Will the Real Healer Please Take a Bow." Miller, Rachel. Co-published simultaneously in *Social Work with Groups* (The Haworth Social Work Practice Press, an imprint of The Haworth Press. Inc.) Vol. 25, No. 1/2, 2002. pp. 65-72; and: *Stories Celebrating Group Work: It's Not Always Easy to Sit on Your Mouth* (ed: Roselle Kurland, and Andrew Malekoff) The Haworth Social Work Practice Press, an imprint of The Haworth Press, Inc., 2002, pp. 65-72. Single or multiple copies of this article are available for a fee from The Haworth Document Delivery Service [1-800-HAWORTH, 9:00 a.m. - 5:00 p.m. (EST). E-mail address: getinfo@haworthpressinc.com].

65

my previous clients with personality disorder. In fact, what I did see quite frequently was a quiet kind of support and caring these so seriously ill patients were able to give each other. Over time I began to wonder if it was the illness that was narcissistic, not the person. What I mean by this is that when people have any life threatening illness, they need all their resources to take care of themselves. Thus, people hearing voices and filled with fear due to delusions or confusion retreat into themselves and have great difficulty connecting to others. This is not a narcissistic personality, but a result of and reaction to a severe illness. Once I was clear on this, I was able to begin to draw upon the real personalities of my group members.

Though many of the young people I treat have good recoveries, the events of the day that clarified my perspective involved two young people who were still experiencing serious symptoms. Pete was a tall black young man who had stopped his medication and was rehospitalized with delusions, hallucinations and manic symptoms. He had been in the hospital for six weeks when the doctor reluctantly allowed me to take him out for a grounds walk. Honestly, I was worried because he had been so violent a few weeks earlier. At that time ten health care workers had to restrain him, but he desperately needed to get out now. He contracted not to run away, and I trusted him to keep his word as he had always done so in the past. He was so down, so very sad at having a relapse when he had been absolutely certain he would be strong enough to conquer this illness without medication.

As we walked around the campus of the hospital we talked. It was a cool winter day so we did not run into many other people, patients or staff. But as we walked past the tall glass windows of the day hospital, someone began waving excitedly. Then she burst out the front doors. It was Simone, a young woman whose symptoms, delusions about a man in a store who talked to her continuously, never responded to treatment, not to Prolixin, Risperdal, Olanzapine, Clozapine, or electro convulsive therapy. She went directly to Pete, saying, "Oh Pete, it's so good to see you." Her hug was as sincere as her words. He seemed to grow taller as his sadness was transformed into joy. They were friends from group, in their own way real friends, and her words and gestures told him how important he was to her. The tears each of us cried at that moment were of love. There was no narcissism in the air that cool day.

From that day on, I knew that the group was to be a safe place, a place of empathy and connections. Forget the books and lectures. Rethink Yalom. There were stages of group development my patients would never reach and that was just fine. These young people needed one place where they could talk about what it means to be diagnosed with schizophrenia, where they could learn about their illness, where they could question their treatment and where they could openly discuss their recent terrifying symptoms. After all, how many people can really understand what it means to say, "I used to think my mother wanted to poison me." For still other patients, the group would be the only place they could relearn how to make eye contact, small talk, or simple human connections.

To create such a group atmosphere required staying focused on the group members' strengths. Some clinicians might say such severely ill patients have few strengths, that they are the least functional with the lowest level of ego functioning. Yet I had experienced so many moments of strength by group members. Stop for a moment and imagine the courage it takes to accept and deal with an illness so stigmatizing and "hopeless." They somehow found the strength to do this, especially together as a group. They had the ability to share their own harrowing experiences with those more recently ill patients. Then there was the group's strength in confronting members' noncompliance or use of substances. The capacity to project hope to new members and take it back into themselves in the process went against all my expectations. And the empathy they could demonstrate with one another often brought me to wonder at the ability of humans to care and love, even in the worst circumstances. With their strength mine also grew. I became increasingly able to experiment and explore new means to guide them. My own hopefulness for them grew.

Slowly I began to break more rules. First, I noticed that patients who had the opportunity to experience group treatment appeared to drop out of treatment less frequently (Miller and Mason, 2001). This led to my changing the treatment strategy so that patients began joining the already scheduled day hospital group sessions while still inpatient. In this way, we guaranteed that patients would have some group experience no matter what the treatment disposition following discharge. Anyone who works in a large hospital knows this meant fighting the system; after all the inpatient, day hospital and outpatient clinic were uniquely separate divisions with little interface. At first I needed permission, but now, two years later, the group has become part of the system. In fact, the inpatient staff's perception of it is so good we might get complaints if we tried to end it.

From the first, I watched to see what worked to make the group a useful experience for the patients. It appeared that anything that made them feel connected helped them feel more hopeful. However, the severity of illness made the usual interaction extraordinarily difficult for many patients. Group activities seemed to help and one by one became part of the group culture. Today, the day hospital/inpatient group begins each morning with a wake-up game of beach ball in which the group works together to keep the ball aloft. The same group ends with a round of stretches followed by three deep breaths. The concept for going around the group with stretches originated with a patient who led us in a round robin of dancing at our second annual Halloween party. The patients also have a ritual round of checking for medication compliance, a "symptom check," and a substance abuse check when needed. This not only encourages their individual and group responsibilities but helps them practice their communication skills.

There are many opportunities for group activities that tap the patients' humanity. It's silly, they laugh, but so enjoy when the group sings happy birthday with a doughnut or Junior Mint with a candle atop. When someone moves from inpatient to day hospital or outpatient, it is marked by "For S/he is a Jolly Good Fellow." Special occasions may merit a pizza party, music and a round of dancing in follow-the-leader format. Making a shower for a soon to be new mother (the doctor) or for a group member's wedding or new apartment usually requires more guidance, but normalizes and fosters pride. Every occasion is an opportunity to be seized and used.

More and more, we tapped the strengths of individual patients. Some patients sang beautifully, danced or drew. Group artists led us to explore mood through color and drawing. They filled the walls of our room with pictures and decoration. Dancers guided us to make our parties great fun. Singers and musicians made Friday's end of week groups so special that we went from awful attendance to near perfect attendance. One member's poetry hangs on the group room wall to continue to help new patients to discuss the trauma of their first hospitalization.

Perhaps the greatest feat for thirty-five of our patients was when they came together to work on a book for other patients, *So They Say I Have Schizophrenia* (Miller and Mason, in print). The group gave of themselves in the hopes of helping other people like themselves. They worked in small groups to brainstorm the book's focus and the elements to be included. Many patients came in on their own time, again and again, to proof read, edit, write chapter introductions, and draw illustrations. It took great courage to expose themselves as they revealed their stories of illness, hospitalization and their difficulties coming to grips with a diagnosis of schizophrenia. They were smart, honest and courageous. I truly believe they could only do this because of their trust in each other's support.

Each year we try new experiments. Now patients are welcome to drop in to visit their old groups simply to say hello. Healthier patients come in to advise and share their firsthand experience of getting well. Patients move almost seamlessly from group to group as their schedules require so that they can move into jobs and school; they are able to plan around health instead of around illness. Patients who were not prepared to leave the daily day hospital symptom management group could stay with that group even when they left the day program for once a week outpatient care. Bit by bit, the groups became one larger community of peers. If they did not know each other well, they knew of each other. We began to make holiday or goodbye parties to include all patients instead of individual groups *and they came.*

Like a healthy family, they (and I) learned to be flexible and creative in order to nurture each other. We had groups of two and groups of twelve. Some patients attended the group each week, some two groups a week, and others once a month. The once a month patients (due to distance or scheduling) did not drop out, and the every week patients did not get angry. They were working together, rooting for each other, spurred on by each other's accomplishments, and supportive in times of failure. When a peer was hospitalized, they visited. Some patients had remarkable recoveries while others struggled. But they did not do it alone.

When I look back to the beginning of my work with my first episode patients, I recognize the importance of using each patient's individual talents, but the real strength, the one that makes the group special, is the ability of members to care for one another. Now I see this so clearly; but in the beginning my focus was on solving each one's unique problems while somehow building cohesion. The problems were overwhelming at times, but staying focused on the cohesion appears to be the key to what I was able to learn later about empathy and caring among first episode clients. I recall clearly my very first group of first episode patients. We had been working together for many months when the hospital made a new–and short-lived–rule requiring patients to be seen in group only. One of the group member's parents had died in Egypt, and the patient, unable to return to mourn with her family, was becoming depressed. At the end of our discussion, the group decided that the patient needed to be seen individually and directed me to "tell the boss that this was absolutely necessary." There was no envy, no malice, no scapegoating or monopolizing, just simple caring from fragile young people willing to risk using their recently practiced assertiveness skills. And I did go to my boss, and I did see her individually, and she did not have a psychotic relapse.

This ability to tap into the patients' capacity to care for one another became the main focus of my role as group leader. I learned to trust the patients to confront each other when necessary and be kind to one another regularly. My mantra became, "Group communication and cohesion is the most valuable outcome of group. Everything else will follow. Only with this connection to each other can they stay honest about their illness, less fearful to face the future and able to stay in treatment."

Two weeks before writing this, I brought a young man about to move from inpatient to the day program into a nighttime outpatient group, one I hoped he would eventually join. This was very unusual because the group he was meeting was high functioning with many members working or attending school. But I knew he needed what only they could offer: hope. I did not need to prepare the group. They, too, knew what he needed. The group had been there for them when they needed it, and they were now happy to be the healers. The group members welcomed him openly; they noticed but understood his occasional distraction; and they encouraged him to believe he could recover. When he told them he was an inpatient, that he had been hearing voices and experiencing paranoia, they smiled and told him about their own hospitalizations, delusions and hallucinations. Several weeks later, as he prepared to move into outpatient, he told his day hospital group that meeting the patients in the outpatient group, who had been in his situation before and who looked normal and had normal lives now, had meant so very much to him. He said he was ready to move into that group. He was looking forward to being part of the group that had given him hope. One day not far from now he will be the one helping the next new patient, of that I am certain.

Our groups have their share of difficult patients. There are patients who fight treatment. They discontinue their medication and use substances. They might have poor insight because of the illness or have very strong defenses, usually denial. There are patients with severe difficulties with interpersonal relationships, patients who are inappropriate, hypersexual, irritable, monopolizing, grandiose, angry, or who have a variety of other problematic personality traits. At this very time there is a young man who is sexually inappropriate, with no insight, using alcohol and telling us he will do whatever he wants whenever he wants to. He attends the day hospital program, where he comes daily to our group without complaint but only participates in other groups when threatened with expulsion from the program. Some days it is hard on the group members, yet they understand he is influenced by continuing symptoms, and therefore are patient with him. I expect one day he will be able to support others as he is now supported. For the time being, the group is providing him with support to stay in treatment. Sometimes that is all we can hope for.

When I need rejuvenation, I think of Tom. Three years after completing treatment with the first episode team, Tom came by to say hello and to ask how some of his old group members were doing. He had been a particularly difficult patient who was in restraints for seven days when I had originally joined the team. His denial had been rock hard, his compliance very poor, and his parents ready to send him packing with each relapse, of which there were three. It had been a long battle for him and he had attended many groups with me. When I told him how nice it was to see him, he said he thought it would be good for me to see how well he was doing. He said he knew that sometimes I worried about them (the group members). He could see it on my face. This day he wanted to cheer me up, he said, so I wouldn't give up on my clients. "I know sometimes we are very tough to work with." His timing was exquisite, better than mine ever could be. The latest recruits to the study were wearing me thin, at times making me feel hopeless. I needed the reminder that the hard work of group would eventually bear fruit. Six months later, Tom came by to say he was graduating from college and going to work as a counselor in a boy's school.

Tapping into the group's strength is a dynamic process, one that changes with the introduction of each new member. This means there is no clear set of rules for building a cohesive and therapeutic group. So what is it that I do in groups? I am still learning. I know I provide a feeling of safety. I provide structure and set limits. When necessary I help patients to connect with each other. I teach them about their illness. I facilitate the exploration of their ambivalence to treatment. I act as the group's organizing ego, but only as much as necessary. Then I step back and watch *the real healers* make magic.

REFERENCES

Freud, S. *On Beginning the Treatment. The Complete Psychological Works of Sigmund Freud*. London: Vol. 12, pp. 124-125, Hogarth Press, 1958.

Miller, R. and Mason, S. *So They Say I Have Schizophrenia.* New York: Columbia University Press (in press).

Miller, R. and Mason, S. (1998) Group Work with First Episode Schizophrenia Clients. *Social Work with Groups,* Vol 21 (1/2).

Yalom, I. (1995) *Theory and Practice of Group Psychotherapy.* 3rd ed. USA: Basic Books.

The Power of Group Work with Kids:
Lessons Learned

Andrew Malekoff

The first group I worked with took place just a few years before publication of the first issue of *Social Work with Groups* in 1978. The group was composed of three girls and three boys, all teenagers. It happened somewhere far from where I grew up and before I knew anything about group work. As the years pass, the experience remains fresh in my memory. The lessons learned deepen with each passing year. Following is the story of Los Seis, my first group, and what it taught me.

MY FIRST KIDS' GROUP

I formed my first kids' group when I was a 22-year old Volunteers in Service to America (VISTA) Volunteer. After graduating from Rutgers College in New Jersey, I bounced around from job to job–warehouse-man, bouncer, and roofer, to name a few. I applied to be a New Jersey State Trooper, FBI agent and air conditioning and refrigeration installer/repairman. For one reason or another none of these worked out. A linebacker at Rutgers, I bulked up to 240 pounds and tried out for three professional football teams. I only made it as far as a couple of semi-pro "farm" teams. Although I was lost, something moved me to

[Haworth co-indexing entry note]: "The Power of Group Work with Kids: Lessons Learned." Malekoff, Andrew. Co-published simultaneously in *Social Work with Groups* (The Haworth Social Work Practice Press, an imprint of The Haworth Press, Inc.) Vol. 25, No. 1/2, 2002, pp. 73-86; and: *Stories Celebrating Group Work: It's Not Always Easy to Sit on Your Mouth* (ed: Roselle Kurland, and Andrew Malekoff) The Haworth Social Work Practice Press, an imprint of The Haworth Press, Inc., 2002, pp. 73-86. Single or multiple copies of this article are available for a fee from The Haworth Document Delivery Service [1-800-HAWORTH, 9:00 a.m. - 5:00 p.m. (EST). E-mail address: getinfo@haworthpressinc.com].

send an application to VISTA. I only knew about VISTA in a vague way as the domestic branch of the more popular Peace Corps. I volunteered as a big brother at Rutgers and I loved kids. So I thought I'd give it a try and apply to VISTA. Maybe I could work with kids in some way, I thought. My application must have passed muster with the VISTA honchos, because they offered me a stint in San Francisco or Grand Island, Nebraska. Inexplicably, I chose to hang my hat in the cornfields rather than by the Bay.

Grand Island is located in mid-Nebraska. When I look at a map of the United States, I see Grand Island smack in the center of the country. It was a town of about 25,000 people at the time, mostly white and middle-class. I also remember there being a fair number of German Americans as I recall. The locale was a mix of suburb and farmland. The community that I called home for nearly three years, located in the northeastern corner of Grand Island, was probably 95% Mexican-American with a good number of working poor families.

None of the roads in that part of town were paved. When I first arrived, I roomed with a local family. A short time later I rented a tiny two-bedroom house on the edge of a cornfield. The rent was $100 a month. A few blocks from my house, pig and cattle auctions were held on Mondays and Tuesdays. Living in Nebraska was nothing like my early years growing up in Newark, New Jersey where the landscape was concrete and telephone poles and the closest thing to a cornfield was the corner bakery.

The group I formed in the spring of 1974 included six kids. There were three boys: Danny, Carlos and Marco; and three girls: Lilly, Mariel, and Toni. They ranged in age from 13 to 18. All were first generation Mexican-Americans. They all knew each other well, living in this close-knit place where everybody seemed to know everybody.

The idea to create a group started percolating after I was in town for only a few days. Danny, whose sister's house I was rooming in, hot-wired a car and took it for a joy ride. It was a rainy night. The car spun out of control, crashing into the side of the sheriff's house. Really! I learned later that Danny's father and older brother had done time in the state penitentiary. I saw Danny headed down the same road. In what turned out to be a good financial investment, I kicked in a couple hundred dollars after being asked to contribute to Danny's bail. Although I was only in Grand Island for a short time, living in Danny's sister's house, I was welcomed with open arms. I enjoyed her home-cooked Mexican meals, developed a friendship with her husband, and adored her four young children. Contributing to the bail was more of an intuitive decision than a rational one, the kind of decision that a feeling of family tends to inspire, right or wrong. It was a decision I never regretted.

During the same time I met an 18-year old young woman Mariel, who was soon to become the senior group member. I found out through the grapevine that she had been through drug rehab more than once. I was advised by someone to go to Mariel's home and meet her parents who were described as very conservative. I was warned that there was no way I'd get anywhere with Mariel without her parents' consent.

It was a wonderful lesson. I learned never to cut parents out of the picture. It made sense to me that the parents of these kids would need to trust the gringo stranger who had suddenly appeared in town. Yet, over the years I have met countless colleagues who perceive anxious parents as a thorn in their professional side and use the cloak of confidentiality to factor them out of the helping equation.

One by one I got to know each of the prospective group members and their parents and brothers and sisters and aunts and uncles. Getting to know everyone seemed easy at first. I received many invitations to home cooked Mexican meals. However, accompanying the delicious food and great company were situations that I was totally unprepared for. For instance, there was the time I received a written marriage proposal from one of the group member's cousins. I never considered a dinner invitation in quite the same way after this.

HANGING OUT

I got to know the prospective group members by hanging out in their homes, in the park, on the basketball court, and here and there. The kids were all children of parents who came a generation earlier from Mexico with their parents to work the local beet farms. I also hung out with the adults, often late into the night. I learned something that didn't take any special assessment skills on my part. The alcohol flowed freely in this place.

There was a Latin club in town. Everyone turned out to dance and have a few beers on Fridays after work. It was a family atmosphere and a time for the community to unite, four generations dancing to contemporary and traditional Mexican music. If a newcomer such as myself wanted to be more than a stranger, the Latin club was the place to be.

I gradually began to feel less like a stranger. When I sensed that people had become more comfortable with me I thought it made sense to get a few of the kids together. I thought that forming a club might serve to address some of their needs such as preventing alcohol abuse and strengthening cultural identity. Many elders in the community feared that assimilation was sucking the rich heritage from their children's souls.

I had an idea. The kids loved to dance and listen to music, and *could they dance*. It seemed to me that sitting around and talking rap group style was one thing we could and would do, but that they would probably like doing a lot more than talking. This wasn't, as they say, rocket science. It just made good sense to me to do what they liked, were good at, and might find meaningful and productive.

All these years later I continue to meet colleagues who assign second-class status to groups that dance and sing and laugh and run and jump and play. An air of condescension and professional arrogance often surrounds the use of nonverbal activities in group, especially in those schools and clinical settings where the spoken word rules the day. When the activity of the group is other than earnest and insightful discussion, parents, referral sources, administrators, and colleagues too often arch a collective eyebrow of disapproval as if to say, "This is nice but when does the real work begin." There is nothing more deadly to the creative process needed to grow good groups than such uninformed, blind, authoritarian rigidity. *Spiritual incarceration*. That is what I call it.

LEARNING FROM THE INSIDE-OUT

As the kids' group took shape, I worried that I didn't know anything about Mexican culture. I decided that the dance floor at the Latin club was a good place to start. The most spirited dances were communal, young and old circling the floor as a large group, accenting the need to stay connected in the present by preserving the past.

If I could learn Mexican dance at the Latin club, I figured that there had to be others in town who could teach me and the group other things we needed to know. I thought that if I could find such people and get to know them that I could convince them to help me, help us.

I didn't know anything about alcoholism either. So I found out about an alcoholism program across the street from the cattle auction. I got to know Jim, the director of the center. We spent some time together and he provided me with literature on the subject. Jim told me that he was in recovery and invited me to an open AA meeting. I didn't know what "recovery" meant, so he taught me. He agreed to help in any way he could. I also met an elementary school teacher who lived in the community. Dolores was a dynamic woman with a great smile, unlimited knowledge about her heritage, boundless energy and a burning desire to help the young people in the community. She was dying to help out. I told her about the group and she agreed to teach dance and sprinkle in some history lessons along the way.

Soon I met others who, as they learned about the group and its purpose, wanted to pitch in too. There were women who offered to sew traditional dresses for the girls to dance in, men who loaned their cherished sombreros to the boys, people in recovery willing to talk about alcoholism and the road to sobriety, and so on. Soon the group had a small army of helpers. And all I had to do was ask.

GIVING UP CONTROL

And so I made another valuable discovery. And this was a big one. I learned that I didn't have to control everything. I could depend on others–others being the kids themselves and the grown ups who had a stake in them. This took a lot of pressure off of me. It meant that I didn't have to know everything. I did have to be willing to trust others and have faith in what they might have to offer. I later discovered that this was a very unpopular way to think among colleagues who revere a one-to-one medical model, where professional is knowledgeable decision maker, client is passive recipient, pathology rules, and DSM is the holy bible. ("Hallelujah," cried the lonely managed care clerk from his desolate outpost in the hinterlands of Corporate America.)

We decided on a group name: *Los Seis*–The Six. As I got to know *Los Seis* better, I realized that despite the overwhelming odds that they faced they had lots to offer. They were attractive, creative, talented, intelligent, energetic, passionate, and open-minded–open minded enough to give me the priceless and timeless gift of letting me into their lives so that I can share this gift, and all I learned from it, with others. Others like you, the reader.

The group met several times a week. It was fun, exciting, and at times puzzling. One day a newspaper crew came to cover the story of the group. As the photographer readied for the shoot, the group unraveled before my eyes. A simmering dispute between Marco and Toni exploded. In frustration, everyone threatened to quit the group. Several ran from the building. I chased them down and persuaded them to return. The full page spread of photos that appeared two days later in the

Sunday paper was so impressive that no reader could have picked up on the chaos that transpired just moments before the photos were taken.

The kids always seemed to bounce back from adversity in the group. But there was more at work than individual resiliency. The group had become a force, a distinct entity with an identity and life of its own. There was an undeniable path that I couldn't explain and didn't understand at the time. Years later I learned about group culture, group process, and strength-based work and it all started to make some sense.

In time, Los Seis became best known as a dance group that traveled throughout the State spreading a message of cultural pride and alcohol abuse prevention. In a sense they became advocates, extending the bonds of belonging beyond the group itself. A highlight was their first public appearance before a gathering of the local community. One of the poems chosen for the event is an epic of the Mexican-American people, the most famous poem of the Chicano movement in America. It's called "I am Joaquin" or "Yo soy Joaquin," written by Rodolfo "Corky" Gonzales (1967), long involved in the civil and human rights movement of the Mexican-American people. The book length poem gave voice to what many in the community felt.

As the lights were turned down in the community center, the group members took turns reading by candlelight as a hundred of their family and friends, young and old, looked on and listened.

I am Joaquin,
Lost in a world of confusion,
caught up in the whirl of a
gringo society,
confused by the rules,
scorned by attitudes,
suppressed by manipulation,
and destroyed by modern society.
My fathers
have lost the economic battle
and won
the struggle of cultural survival . . . (p. 6)
La Raza!
Mejicano!
Espanol!
Latino!
Hispano!
Chicano!

or whatever I call myself,
I look the same
I feel the same
I cry
and
sing the same
I am the masses of my people and
I refuse to be absorbed.
I am Joaquin.
The odds are great
but my spirit is strong,
my faith unbreakable,
my blood is pure.
I am Aztec prince and Christian Christ.
I shall endure!
I will endure! (pp. 98-99)

Working with Los Seis has been one of the enduring pleasures of my life. Nevertheless, at the time I couldn't help but wonder, how did this happen? What did I do to help make it happen? Was it a fluke? Could I do it again?

EARLY LESSONS AND ENDURING PRINCIPLES

It has been 28 years since Los Seis and my belief in the value of good group experiences for kids has only grown despite countless obstacles. In time I became a student, and then a teacher and author, of what was at first the product of an intuitive journey. As I continued the journey, later in graduate school and then in agency work, I became disheartened to see so many talented people bailing out and abandoning group work with kids. But who could blame them? Higher education, with a few notable exceptions, has failed. And there is little or no reliable support and supervision in most work places.

Much of what passes as group work these days is nothing more than curriculum-driven pseudo group work with little interaction amongst group members, no mutual aid, cookbook agendas, and canned exercises. The emphasis is on controlling kids, shoving education down their throats, and stamping out spontaneity and creativity.

Somewhere along the way I became a missionary of sorts, encouraging others to stay the course and attempting to demystify group work so that it could be more easily understood and purposefully practiced.

And so, with the spirit of Los Seis in mind and heart, I'll conclude with seven principles and a poem that I hope you will embrace, seven strength-based bricks accompanied by a lyrical message to begin building a foundation for the important work ahead: I hope that . . .

- those of you who work with young people in groups or who administer programs that include group work, will learn that a group shouldn't be formed on the basis of a diagnosis or label. I want you to be crystal clear that a group should be formed on the basis of particular needs that the group is being pulled together to address. Felt needs are different that ascribed labels. Understanding need is where we begin in group work. Such a simple concept, yet so foreign to so many.

- you will learn to structure your groups to invite the whole person and not just the troubled or hurt or broken parts. There is so much talk these days about strengths and wellness. This is hardly a new and revolutionary concept. But it has been neglected for too long. However, good group work practice has been paying attention to people's strengths since the days of the original settlement houses over 100 years ago, mostly without any fanfare.

- you will value the use of verbal and non-verbal activities and will, for once and for all, learn to relax and to abandon the strange and bizarre belief that the only successful group is one that consists of young people who sit still and speak politely and insightfully.

- you will come to understand that losing control is not where you want to get away from, it's where you want to get to. What I mean by this is, when control is turned over to the group and when the group worker gives up his or her centrality in the group, that mutual aid can follow and then members can find the expression they have to offer. Encouraging "what they have to offer"–that's the kind of group work we need to practice, that's what real empowerment is all about.

- you will stay tuned in to the near things and far things, the near things of individual need and the far things of social reform. Our young group members need to see the potential of changing not only oneself but also one's surroundings, so that they may become active participants in community affairs, so that they might make a difference, might change the world one day where we have failed to. A good group can be a great start for this kind of consciousness development and action among young people.

- you will learn that anxious and angry parents are not our enemies and that we must collaborate with them and form stable alliances with them if we are to be successful with their children. Many parents suffer from profound isolation and self-doubt. We must learn to embrace their frustration and anxiety rather than become defensive and rejecting. They get enough of that as it is.
- you will learn that a good group has a life of its own, each one with a unique personality—what we group workers refer to as a culture. We must learn to value the developmental life of a group. Because if people can take this from today, when those who inhabit the world outside of our groups question the value of our efforts, amidst the noise and movement and excitement of typical kids groups—and when they raise an eyebrow or toss puzzled and disapproving looks our way and ask us, "What is going on in there?!", we'll have more confidence to move ahead and to hang in there and not bail out as too many an adult already has.

I'll leave you with a poem (see below) that I wrote on the existential plight of those of us who work with kids in groups and the faith that is needed to stay the course. The poem, which I wrote while watching a group of kids in a roller rink, is my attempt to demystify the concept of group process (Malekoff, 1997).

WHAT IS GOING ON IN THERE?: QUESTION AND RESPONSE

What is going on in There? (The question)

We bring our kids to you,
To see what you can do;

They meet a bunch of others,
See, we are all their mothers;
We hear a ton of noise,
And, yes, boys will be boys (and girls will be girls);

But what is going on in there?,
Nothing much we fear.

Our rooms are side by side,
And it's not my style to chide;

But your group's a bit too crazy.
And what you're doing's kind of hazy;

After all they're here to talk,
Yet all they do is squeal and squawk;

What is going on in there?
Nothing much we fear.

Hi I'm from the school,
And it's not my style to duel;

But Johnny's in your group,
And I know that you're no dupe;

But his dad has called on me,
To gain some clarity;

So what is going on in there?,
Nothing much, I fear.

Now here we are alas,
Facing you in masse;

We haven't got all day,
So what have you to say;

About this thing called group,
This strange and foggy soup;

Just what is going on in there?,
Nothing much, we fear.
What is Going on in There? (The Response)

If you
really
wish to
know,

have a
seat,
don't plan
to go.

It will
take
awhile
to get,
but you
will
get it,
so
don't you
fret.

A group
begins
by building
trust,
chipping ways
at the
surface crust.

Once
the uneasy
feeling is
lost,
a battle rages
for who's
the boss;
Kings and
Queens
of what's
okay
and who
shall
have the
final say.

Once that's

clear
a moment
of calm,
is quickly
followed
by the
slapping of
palms.

A clan
like feeling
fills
the air,
the sharing
of joy,
hope,
and despair.

Family
dramas
are replayed,
so new
directions
can be
made.

Then in
awhile
each
one
stands out,
confident
of his
own
special
clout.

By then
the group has
discovered
its

pace,
a secret gathering
in a special place.

Nothing
like it
has occurred
before,
a bond
that exist
beyond
the door.

And
finally
it's time
to say
good-bye,
a giggle,
a
tear,
a
hug,
a
sigh.

Hard to
accept,
easy to
deny,
the
group
is gone
yet
forever
alive.

So you've
asked me
"what is
going

on in
there?,"
I hope
that my
story has
helped
make it
clear.

Maybe
now
it is
easier
to see,
that a
group
has a
life,
just
like
you
and
like
me.

AUTHOR NOTE

This narrative is adapted from an article that appeared in *Families in Society* (May-June, 2001, 82: 3) entitled: "The Power of Group Work with Kids: A Practitioner's Reflection on Strengths-Based Practice," 243-249.

REFERENCES

Gonzales, R. (1967). *I Am Joaquin.* New York: Bantam.
Malekoff, A. (1997). *Group Work with Adolescents: Principles and Practice.* New York: Guilford, 50-52.

If Only They Were Adults
My Job Would Be Easier

Cynthia G. Cavallo

There is a misconception about group work with children and youth that I encountered midway through my career. While at Youth Directions and Alternatives, a small youth agency on suburban Long Island, New York, one of my staff members with whom I worked intensely around the "chaos" he was experiencing in his group blurted out one day, "If only they were adults my job would be easier." This worker was an MSW. I tried diligently to bring him to a place where he could understand the dynamics of group work with adolescents. However, he struggled throughout the group and could not see the gains his clients were making. He just felt things were "out of control." This particular worker never did develop a comfort level with his role as group facilitator and eventually moved on to a different position within a year of being hired.

My first professional group work experience was at a Settlement House in the Bronx, NY. I was hired, after completing my graduate degree from Teachers College of Columbia University in Family and Community Education, to facilitate groups for parents of newborns. I came to the position with limited group work experience. As I started out, I found myself feeling lost and confused in the groups. I was fortunate to be supervised by someone with a strong belief and significant training in group work. The weekly supervision, process recordings and overall support were extremely beneficial. I was given the opportunity to share my frustrations and fears and critically analyze my work in a

[Haworth co-indexing entry note]: "If Only They Were Adults My Job Would Be Easier." Cavallo, Cynthia G. Co-published simultaneously in *Social Work with Groups* (The Haworth Social Work Practice Press, an imprint of The Haworth Press, Inc.) Vol. 25, No. 1/2, 2002, pp. 87-92; and: *Stories Celebrating Group Work: It's Not Always Easy to Sit on Your Mouth* (ed: Roselle Kurland, and Andrew Malekoff) The Haworth Social Work Practice Press, an imprint of The Haworth Press, Inc., 2002, pp. 87-92. Single or multiple copies of this article are available for a fee from The Haworth Document Delivery Service [1-800-HAWORTH, 9:00 a.m. - 5:00 p.m. (EST). E-mail address: getinfo@haworthpressinc.com].

supportive, non-judgmental atmosphere. It always helped me to throw myself back into the group the following week!

Eventually I ended up as Executive Director of Youth Directions and Alternatives. The foundation of that agency was group work. I found myself with a young, highly dedicated and energetic staff that had little if no experience and/or training in group work (let alone group work with youth). In many ways it felt like we were shooting in the dark. Many of the groups we ran were in host settings–mainly school buildings, creating a situation where tensions sometimes ran high between my staff, who rolled with the groups, and the school staff, who viewed the groups as successful if all of the students were quietly sitting in their seats and calmly discussing their "issues." It was not uncommon for me to receive phone calls from someone at the School district complaining about the noise and/or level of activity coming from the room in which the group met. I always knew we were doing good work. It was obvious to me from the relationship our staff was able to establish with the very high-risk youth with whom we worked. I often found this situation to be frustrating for me as a supervisor. It often required a meeting between our staff and school district staff in order to rectify the situation. But I somehow always left feeling that I was not able to convey clearly enough the importance of the work that was being accomplished in the groups.

Then one day a brochure came across my desk advertising a multi-session training on facilitation of groups for youth. It was extremely appealing to me, given the struggles I was experiencing as a supervisor and therefore I signed up for the training. Andy Malekoff of North Shore Child and Family Guidance Center, a mental health agency located on Long Island, was offering it. It proved to be one of the most valuable trainings I ever attended. It helped to give me a strong basis for the work my agency was doing, validated that work and catapulted me forward in my belief that groups for youth, if handled properly, could be a powerful catalyst for change. For instance, the notion that chaos in groups with youth was normal and expected gave me a great sense of relief. This training also helped me to identify the "work" that was being accomplished through the chaos. A group of noisy youth who are tossing a sponge around the room while talking about their issues are using the sponge as a way of connecting and relating to one another. They are not tossing it around in order to be outrageous or annoy the facilitator. I began to find better ways to explain the work so others could understand it.

This training gave me the tools to support my staff in their work and to articulate that work to those who were collaborating with us. My staff and I suddenly felt empowered enough to stand by our convictions because we had a framework from which to explain our work. We were better able to resist the temptation to cave in when people reported that the group appeared to be unproductive, foolish or out of control. For instance, a group of acting out teens who come together weekly in a group may use board games as a mechanism for them to join together–become part of something greater than themselves in a school setting. It can help them to establish a sense of belonging, provide a way to practice cooperating with their peers and provide them with a chance to become part of a team (something they may not have been able to master prior to this). An activity often provides a less stressful way for youth to engage in conversation with one another as well. We now had the tools to explain that the chaos and activity was part of the process and the youth who were participating were gaining from the experience.

My new found enthusiasm around group work became obvious to my colleagues and I was asked to expand my training role beyond my own staff to include group work training for all youth workers in our town Youth Bureau system. Additionally, I provided some training to outside systems as well. Expanding training in this area not only helped me assist others to grow professionally in their work, it also illustrated to me the great need for training in this area at undergraduate and graduate level programs.

In one case, I was asked to provide training on group work with children and youth to a group of Guidance Counselors at a local school district. One particular participant projected a strong sense of resistance to the training and had very little to offer during the first half of the day. During the second half of the day he revealed that he had once facilitated a group for high risk, disenfranchised boys in the high school. The boys met with him weekly during their lunch hour. This counselor experienced the groups as chaotic and non-productive and felt nothing was happening so he eventually disbanded the group. After he shared this information I suggested that he might consider the fact that these disconnected, acting out boys who never participated in any school activities *showed up*–during their lunch hour–each week. This in and of itself, was an accomplishment and disbanding the group because of the facilitator's feelings of "chaos" hindered his ability to acknowledge to the boys what they *were* able to accomplish. I pointed out that getting these youth to attend a group on a regular basis tapped into their strengths. If they felt safe enough to do this he could have built on it by creating a greater sense of belonging and competence for these boys. He lost the opportunity to work with these boys in a meaningful, supportive way.

Four years ago, I became the Executive Director of The Coalition On Child Abuse and Neglect, a non-profit organization on suburban L.I. This is an agency which began as a coalition of organizations that addressed the issue of abuse and neglect; however, the agency was beginning to grow and to include direct service programs. Upon meeting one of my staff members for the first time, she indicated to me that she was eager to start groups for children who had been sexually abused. She had been working for several years with these children and their non offending parents and siblings individually through the agency's Child Victim Advocate Program and saw the great need for groups that would help to break down the isolation these families were experiencing and provide them with additional support. Unbeknownst to her, she was speaking to someone who could not agree with her more! I was thrilled to be able to bring group work with youth to my new agency as well as to the population we served. Less than a year later, we began our group work program–Project Kidz Talk–for this population. It includes activity/discussion groups for the child victim and their non-offending siblings and a simultaneous discussion group for the non-offending parent(s). We started the project on a shoestring budget, utilizing agency fundraised money. That was three years ago. Today the project has ongoing support with a budget of over $50,000 and we recently received start up funds to expand into a neighboring county.

Our planning for this program included the development of a training program for staff and interns involved in the program, outreach to and orientation of group members, dialogue with therapists involved with our clients as well as the governmental systems working with these families such as Child Protective Services, Law Enforcement and the District Attorney's Office. These discussions did not always go smoothly. We found some service providers resistant to our work. In one case, while meeting with a field work supervisor from a local university whose intern was involved in the facilitation of our groups, she requested that we not assign the intern to the young children's groups since it was not a good use of interns to "baby sit." As we expand the program in to another county, we are finding resistance to the program from those who prosecute the children's cases. One person indicated to us that she was reluctant to allow us to "throw victims together." She felt it would negatively affect the outcome of the case. Ironically, what we have found in doing this work is that it actually supports a positive outcome for these cases. When supporting victims and their families, they are better able to successfully negotiate and follow through with the systems that investigate and prosecute. I find that we continually need to educate those in and out of the profession regarding the value of group work with children and youth. It has become part of the "work" for me.

When I reflect on this program I am proud to have been a part of it. The project won an entrepreneur of the year award in 1999 for a booklet the children developed preparing other children for the court process. The children's individual therapists reported that the group process had helped these children progress in their individual therapy. Toward the end of the first round of groups, one of the group facilitators had the children share how they felt about being part of it. One little five-year-old girl who had not spoken very much through the groups raised her hand. She told the group that she was glad that she had participated in the program because she "doesn't feel purple in a white world any more." Nothing else needs to be said.

I have also found that our group work program is not only beneficial to those it serves, it has been very beneficial to the agency as a whole. I love talking about this program, I believe in the work. As Executive Director it provides me with talking points that funders and donors can understand. I can share with them the projects the children work on, feedback from the children's individual therapists as well as statements that have come out of the groups. For instance, I served as facilitator of the very first parents group. During one of the final weeks we were discussing how the group had benefited the moms who attended. One mom, whose daughter's case of sex abuse had been going on for several years, stated that she felt as if she has been mourning the death of her daughter's childhood all of these years and she didn't want to feel as if she was at a funeral for the rest of her life! She felt the support she gained from the group was helping her to move away from the "funeral." Also, almost everyone has experienced being part of a group at some point in their lives, so when discussing this service with people who might be interested in supporting us, it brings it to "life" for them. They can think about groups they might have been involved in and how they supported them. It was an unexpected benefit of the program that it makes my job easier to "sell" the agency to those who are able to support our efforts.

I still believe there is a lot of work ahead of us. I have not yet seen undergraduate or graduate students coming to us prepared with the understanding and skills necessary to implement successful group work services for children and youth, even though many new graduates find themselves responsible for providing such a service in their initial professional positions. I have not yet seen a commitment on the part of training institutions to make this a priority. It leaves those of us in the field with the responsibility to provide on-the-job training to those we hire, a commitment I am willing to make. I am willing to make it because I have seen the power of groups. I have seen disenfranchised youth and sexually abused children move to healthier places in their lives because of the group work process. And secondarily, I have seen the power of groups benefit an agency as a whole, bringing it to life for its supporters!

Pitfalls, Pratfalls, Shortfalls and Windfalls: Reflections on Forming and Being Formed by Groups

Ann Rosegrant Alvarez

INTRODUCTION

Two young apple trees stand in the side yard. Purchased and planted on the same day, they could be expected to look and act the same. They do not. One has grown straight, with limbs branching out symmetrically along the trunk. This year, for the first time, it produced a bountiful crop of apples. The other tree, however, has not thrived. Early on, it had a tendency to lean. Its planters did not have the resources, knowledge, time or energy to help redirect its growth, but relied on a makeshift method that may have exacerbated the problem. Located farther from the faucet, it received less water than the other sapling. Additional factors are less obvious, but certainly differing locations result in differing amounts of sunlight, wind and rain, and it is clear that winter-starved deer and rabbits supplemented their diet with the bark of the flawed tree. Pouring all its energy into sheer survival, this tree produced no more than a few undersized apples this year. Judging by its gnarled and twisted shape, bug-infested leaves, uneven limbs, and the ulcerated crater near its base, no better yield can be expected from it in the future.

[Haworth co-indexing entry note]: "Pitfalls, Pratfalls, Shortfalls and Windfalls: Reflections on Forming and Being Formed by Groups." Alvarez. Ann Rosegrant. Co-published simultaneously in *Social Work with Groups* (The Haworth Social Work Practice Press, an imprint of The Haworth Press, Inc.) Vol. 25, No. 1/2, 2002, pp. 93-105; and: *Stories Celebrating Group Work: It's Not Always Easy to Sit on Your Mouth* (ed: Roselle Kurland, and Andrew Malekoff) The Haworth Social Work Practice Press, an imprint of The Haworth Press, Inc., 2002, pp. 93-105. Single or multiple copies of this article are available for a fee from The Haworth Document Delivery Service [1-800-HAWORTH, 9:00 a.m. - 5:00 p.m. (EST). E-mail address: getinfo@haworthpressinc.com].

93

Some of the factors that have contributed to these trees' differential growth and productivity are obvious, while others are not. Clearly, though, early events and intervention have had an ongoing impact on their development. In this respect, we can draw parallels between questions and assumptions about the apple trees and about groups. What explains differences among groups? What contributes to different outcomes? Sometimes it is what we, as facilitators, do; other times, it may be what we don't do. In any case, much of the outcome is heavily influenced by the early stages of group development—what has been termed the "forming" stage.

This stage includes many aspects, including setting up the physical environment, creating an atmosphere of safety, sharing and agreeing upon group purpose and goals, and beginning to develop ways of interacting together according to shared norms. While these aspects may vary in timing and sequencing, they can be expected in groups led by social workers. These groups include therapy groups, support groups, task groups and learning groups.

I have worked for agencies and organization with groups, sometimes toward therapeutic goals. In recent years, however, my group work has been primarily with educational groups in classrooms, workshops, and trainings. The stages of group development are still pertinent in these settings, and the "forming" segment can affect subsequent interactions and productivity powerfully and, sometimes, irreversibly.

As a social work educator, I have chosen to focus this paper on the early, or forming, stages of classroom learning groups. It is important to note that, for the past ten years, the courses I will reference have *not* been framed as group work courses. Rather, they have been in the areas of macro social work, and often, specifically, community practice. It has been my experience that in these courses, students do not necessarily expect to learn about groups, and may even be resistant to such learning. Odd though it may seem to the group worker reader, it often falls to me to persuade the macro students that skills in working with groups will be crucial to their professional development, and that our classroom activities will be transferable to the field.

I have a great deal of experience with these classroom groups, having participated in them as a student for decades and as a teacher for nearly that long. Moreover, they are interesting to compare with other groups, displaying some features in common and some that are specific to them. For example, the group facilitator, or teacher, of classroom groups probably has no control over who enrolls in the class, or even how many. The teacher probably has only minimal say, if any, about where the class meets, or what the venue has to offer, in terms of either facilities or location relative to important considerations such as parking, previous or subsequent classes, day care, students' home locations, etc. The class is time-limited, and therefore will have somewhat predictable developmental stages. It also requires a certain pace and does not allow for extreme variation in the ultimate outcome. Students who take the class can fall anywhere on a continuum of voluntary to involuntary participation; some may have chosen to take it, and exhibit great enthusiasm, while others may view the course as an unpalatable requirement. Clearly, this has implications for involvement, participation and outcome.

> It is the first day of class, and I have left nothing to chance. I checked out the room ahead of time, assessing AV equipment and placing the room in relation to phone, restrooms and vending machines. I previewed the class list to see if I know any of the students, to check the breakdown by gender, full-time vs. part-time, etc.–and to try to make a solid attempt at correctly pronouncing each student's name. I ordered and/or brought AV materials. I prepared an agenda. I am ready with the syllabus and any additional necessary handouts. I arrive early enough to arrange the chairs in a circle, or to ask the students to do so, and to write the agenda on the board. I follow the order I have set out, and the class runs pretty much as I planned. What could be more straightforward? And yet the actual experience of this session–and the few that immediately follow it, which may roughly constitute the "forming" stage–is as varied as the students in the room. What contributes to this variability? What factors can optimize predictability and success?

In the subsequent sections, I will present and discuss some examples of what I have seen go well or badly in the forming of groups. In these vignettes I will alter details and circumstances to preserve confidentiality. I will discuss my experiences with the early, or forming, stage of classroom learning groups within the following framework: pitfalls, pratfalls, shortfalls and windfalls. These sections will feature examples, based on which the conclusion will summarize important points and my learning related to them. I hope that through my sharing mistakes, as well as successes, readers may be spared some of the growth experiences from which I have doubtless benefited–but would just as soon have missed!

PITFALLS

Kindness and intelligence don't always deliver us from the pitfalls and traps: there are always failures of love, of will, of imagination. There is no way to take the danger out of human relationships.

–Barbara Grizzuti Harrison ("Secrets Women Tell Each Other")
McCall's, 1975

There are myriad challenges to face when planting and nurturing a tree. Similarly, forming a group is subject to many potential and actual problems. One of the biggest problems in trying to set up a course as a learning group–what I also like to call a learning community–is that students' expectations of a class are often very different. Based on what I hear from students and other faculty, I believe that most classes are still taught according to what has been termed the "banking" method, which assumes that knowledge is "owned" by the teacher, and "transferred" to the students during class sessions. This does, indeed, represent a version of a learning group, but it runs counter to my vision of the group as a learning community. My goal in such a context is to create an environment in which students feel safe and competent to share opinions and experiences, to risk error or confrontation, and to collaborate toward achieving both group and individual learning goals.

Students may be not only unfamiliar with such an approach, but actually resistant to it. Many students take some time to accept an experiential and collaborative approach to learning, and may struggle with the concept of their teacher as a co-learner and facilitator, as well as the credibility of their fellow class members as co-teachers. Some, moreover, cannot tolerate it. For example, at the end of the first session of one class, I was buttonholed by a student who interrogated me about my methods. Very seriously and sincerely, she informed me that she did not feel a class was worthwhile unless she came out of each session with approximately twelve pages of notes. When I confirmed her suspicion that she was unlikely to achieve that goal in my class, which would include very little straight lecture, she concluded–and I agreed regretfully–that she would probably be better off in another class. It is likely that she now has the satisfaction of knowing that a file folder in a box somewhere contains extensive notes from another section of that class. She may never have experienced, however, working through the issues with a group of her fellow students.

Communicating to students that the class is to operate as a learning community, and explaining what that means, is therefore one of the first tasks of forming the group. This communication must be both explicit, in the form of written and verbal instructions and description, and implicit–demonstrated in the way the class is set up and conducted. One obvious potential problem with this is that the setting may not be conducive to the goals.

Several years ago I taught a class that was scheduled in a building that was unfamiliar to me and to the students. It was off our normal route, parking options were limited and felt unsafe, and the room itself was totally inhospitable. I never could figure out exactly what its function had been, but it was huge, carpeted in a dismally dark shade of green, and had a raised section at one end that could have been a performance area. In this near-cavern, the ten of us huddled during the winter months of the class tenure, pulling our meager number of chairs off-center, so as to de-emphasize how few of us there were to fill this inappropriately large space. Initially, I tried to get the room assignment changed, but I was not successful. I think that part of the reason I did not persist was that I sank into a feeling of doomed depression engendered by the setting. Every session felt like sleepwalking, or slogging through underwater muck. I should never have ignored my own principles about selecting and setting the environment!

In the beginning stages of a group–learning groups included–it is important for members to learn something about each other. In a class setting, this can include at a minimum: names, any personal or professional experience with the topic, and the reason for being in that specific class. One way to help develop norms of safety and trust from the very beginning is to assure class members that they can be honest, for example, about stating openly that they are only in the class because it is a requirement–and then being careful not to display any negative affect or reaction if that is their response. It is important to recognize that when openness is encouraged, there will be occasional surprises.

In the early sessions of the class, I often begin with a non-interactive round that may be substantive, or may simply be a way to focus the group together and for people to share information about themselves. An icebreaker that I use frequently asks people to name a comfort food and explain its significance to them within their culture/family. One semester this was going along smoothly, with some creative contributions, when the round got to a student I'll call Amanda. Amanda named and described her food, which was unique to her cultural and ethnic heritage, and the class seemed appropriately interested. Things fell apart, however, when Amanda did–blurting out that her mother knew this was her favorite food, and served it to her only to soothe her feelings at special times . . . for example, after having beaten her and then locked her up in the closet for hours. This was a lot for the class to handle during what seemed like an innocuous introductory exercise, and at an early point in the semester. This revelation and dealing with it reminded me that each participant and every group is unique, and nothing will ever work exactly the same from one group to another; it is necessary and important to expect the unexpected, and a facilitator cannot afford to become complacent or inattentive.

We all occasionally meet unusual challenges, such as those related to the tragic terrorist attack of the U.S. on September 11, 2001. For many schools, this event came at the semester's beginning, or the forming stage of the learning community. Many of us struggled to balance process and task appropriately, and to allow time for students (and teachers) to vent, rage, grieve, and mourn–while moving forward with the semester's learning goals. Of course, a primary tenet of group work indicates that *not* dealing with the emotional content would, in any case, have prevented the group from effectively engaging with the intellectual content.

PRATFALLS

Mistakes are a fact of life. It is the response to error that counts.

–Nikki Giovanni *(Black Feeling/Black Talk/Black Judgement,* 1970)

It is with wry humility that a gardener confesses to having killed a young tree by "fertilizing" it with poison, or–perhaps more in the spirit of a "pratfall"–by accidentally slashing it in the act of falling, after tripping with an ax while intending to lop off one small limb. Sometimes our best efforts as gardeners or as group leaders go awry. Determined to avoid the mistakes of an earlier group, for example, we may overcompensate with the current one. Feedback from our student group members may lead us to modify our approach in response to idiosyncratic perceptions or evaluations, rather than trusting our own instincts.

> One semester, discussions were dominated by a student who took way too much air time and was very difficult to rein in, even though I used multiple forms and occasions for intervention. Subsequent evaluations reflected the discomfort the rest of the class had felt with this situation. The next semester, during the first round of introductions during the first session, one young woman went on at considerable length. She spoke three times as long as anyone else and provided a great deal of unnecessary detail. I wanted to be sure that I gave her a clear message about appropriate participation and that the rest of the class also had faith that I would be monitoring for equitable contributions. At the end of the introductions, therefore, I made some strong and pointed comments about self-monitoring, and being careful that the timing and length of remarks were on target. The young woman turned out to have bi-polar syndrome, and–possibly because her faith in her ability to judge her own appropriateness was shaken–my comments had the effect of silencing her for most of the rest of the semester. The rest of the class, too, was negatively affected; instead of making other members feel safe, my comments had made them wary of making their own contributions. My attempt to be helpful and sensitive to the group thus had a chilling impact on the class, and the power of the facilitator was demonstrated forcefully to me.

SHORTFALLS

> *Aim at heaven and you will get earth thrown in. Aim at earth and you will get neither.*

> –C. S. Lewis *(Mere Christianity,* 1952)

Sometimes a harvest–or a group–just does not live up to expectations. We may think we have done everything right, but the end result is somehow less than it should be. After planting according to the book, watering faithfully, and pruning ruthlessly, the blossoms may not be pollinated, the fruit may have worms, or it may be shriveled and taste-less. In like manner, despite skilled planning and facilitation from a teacher, sometimes a classroom group may not coalesce.

> One recent semester I had a small class that I could not seem to en-ergize or engage. I tried everything I could think of to try to build a relationship with the class members, both as individuals and as a group, and to encourage participation. However, nothing I did seemed to make a difference; the group remained apathetic, lethar-gic and–to my eyes–uninterested and unmotivated. I concluded that we must have somehow gotten off on the wrong foot; I must have done something in the forming stages to close people off and shut them up. I was, therefore, amazed at the end of the semester to have several students separately confide to me that they had felt more comfortable and safer in my class than any other and, as a re-sult, had participated in it more than any other. Clearly, the stu-dents' expectations differed from mine, and my expectations were coloring my interpretation of the group and their interaction in it. The learning group had apparently been more successful for its members than I had credited it with being; but the results were still disappointing to me.

Another version of a shortfall occurs when teachers, as group lead-ers, do not live up to their own expectations. For most of us, this is the most disappointing version, and these failures may haunt us for a long time. We can only hope and strive to learn from and improve because of them.

> I recall vividly a class session during which I missed an eminently teachable moment. During a warmup, the group was imaging and physically passing energy from one to another. Early on, a hug was passed along, but it morphed into another exchange. When the en-ergy reached two adjacent men friends, one of them tossed off, "Just don't hug me!" This presented a wonderful opportunity to discuss the homophobic implications of the remark, its potential for contributing to a homophobic and heterosexist classroom at-mosphere, and the possible ramifications, both within this class and in other settings. For a variety of reasons–including the stage of group development and the standing in the class of the speaker, who was one of only three males and already noticeable for a ten-dency to offend unintentionally–I chose not to address this re-

mark. I have regretted it ever since, and have always wondered what level of openness and shared growth the class might have achieved if I had followed through with the opportunity to grapple with this issue together.

WINDFALLS

. . . you don't need a weatherman to know which way the wind blows . . .

–Bob Dylan ("Subterranean Homesick Blues," 1965)

Even knowing which way the wind blows may not tell us what it will blow our way. When the wind blows just right, it may knock the apples off the tree–saving the harvesters the trouble of picking them, or providing an unexpected, sweet treat for such passersby as the fox, the deer and the wild turkey. Anyone who has worked with groups must have stories of those unexpected, serendipitous moments when the process and the participants come together to create something far larger than the apparent sum of the parts. In these cases, sometimes the biggest challenge for the facilitator is to step back and let it happen, and not to overprocess it afterward. These moments can occur in the beginning stages of a group, as well as in the later ones. Several examples come to mind.

I often start a semester with a "Multiple Roles" exercise I learned from Beth Glover Reed. This involves students responding to sequenced trigger statements by moving after each is read to a "station" that features the response with which they resonate most strongly. One trigger that often sparks very interesting discussions is, "My biggest concern/fear about the MSW program is that . . ." One possible response, in particular–". . . I will change in ways I don't want to"–elicits a lot of emotion, and the students who go to that station tend to interact in ways that go far deeper than their superficial acquaintance at that point would seem to justify. When the discussion is opened up to the group as a whole, it has led to profound considerations of class, status, relationships and students' perceptions of themselves, as well as how they are perceived within their communities.

A very effective icebreaker and discussion trigger begins with the facilitator's dealing out a deck of cards, each with a "label" attached to it. Participants get five cards each, and pass on to their neighbor first two cards, then one, and then as many as they want to and can persuade someone else to take. This can be very revealing, both of people's biases and what they value. For instance, in a recent group, one woman explained that she had held onto "wheelchair user" after it got passed to her, because that card and identity held no fear for her. For as long as she could remember her mother had been a wheelchair user, and had gone about her life cheerfully and competently. She, therefore, viewed that as a very manageable circumstance–while to others in the group it had seemed insurmountably challenging. This was an important eye-opener for the group–a vivid demonstration of both how and why perspectives may differ, and what impact that may have on people's attitudes and lives.

Interactions that occur later in the life of a group can often be traced back to the early stages. A sense of safety and trust, which may be developed in the forming stage, can bear fruit during subsequent stages. This was no doubt the case with the class during which a mature African-American woman broke into the agenda one session to pose a frustrated query to the group. Why was it, she asked, that in all of her classes, whenever race was discussed, the white students pulled back and left all of the discussion to students of color? While the student was emotional about this, the question was framed in such a way, and the ground had been prepared in such a way, that–once they got over their initial surprise–the other students were able to respond in a thoughtful and non-defensive way. This led to one of the best classroom discussions on race and the general unhelpfulness and sometimes debilitating consequences of "white guilt" in which I have ever participated. In addition, it had special value in my eyes because it was student-initiated, rather than being part of my agenda for the class.

CONCLUSION

So after all this, what have I learned about developing classroom groups into learning communities? Clearly, the forming stage is crucial to this process. Following are some of my thoughts on this topic.

- It is important to communicate expectations clearly and respectfully.
- It is important that the group "buy into" the process, especially since some indeterminate proportion of class members may qualify as "involuntary members." Processes and norms must therefore be explained and developed very explicitly. Some of these, such as collaborative approaches to classroom learning, may be difficult to adopt for students who may have been socialized very differently in the past. I therefore explain both the approach I will use and the rationale for it as clearly as possible.
- It is important to model principles and techniques effectively. In addition, when appropriate, discussion should clarify both what has been done and why, with the explicit goal of helping students transform activities and interactions into possibilities for their own practice. Having previously favored a more subtle approach that did not always ensure the desired outcome, I now focus discussion directly on adaptations and applications that students can make in the future, since otherwise many of them may not make these connections themselves.
- Just as no two individuals are totally alike, no two groups are totally alike. Group facilitators must expect the unexpected, and be prepared to deal with it. Even the most innocent-seeming icebreaker has the potential to be emotionally, mentally or physically challenging to participants.
- Follow your own instincts, and adhere to your own principles! Never allow leader inertia to compromise a classroom group. For example, the room setting I described previously seriously affected the semester in a negative way. Another time, I was assigned a room with chairs bolted down in rows ascending from a podium, auditorium-style. I did persist with a change in venue for this class, and the atmosphere and our process improved immensely.
- While we begin each semester's class with an awareness of our history with it, it is important not to be over-influenced by events or feedback from the most recent past, but to remember the overview of the broader experience.
- The experience of group members is different from that of the facilitator. Their assessment of its strengths and limitations may be different, as well. The use of formative evaluation from the very beginning of a group can help the facilitator track group thoughts, feelings and assessment of the class.

- When possible, it is important to deal with the moment and material as it presents itself. Otherwise, it is at least advisable to return to it rather than to let it go underground.
- The selection of the "right" activity or exercise for the time or stage can help a group move forward. This requires flexibility, as well as a wide repertoire from which to draw. I continue to strive to temper my tendency to overplan with the realization that I may have to jettison all agenda items to attend to a matter that affects group growth and ultimate productivity.
- Trust the process, trust the process, trust the process! When the groundwork has been laid thoughtfully by a skilled and trained facilitator, process and outcomes may vary but should ultimately be a positive reflection of what has been established in the collaborative setting of an authentic learning community. While I have been humbled repeatedly by realizations of my own fallibility and ignorance, I have also experienced moments of grace that have served to keep me going–and coming back for more.

These are only some of the possible gleanings from my experiences forming classroom groups. As with much group work, many of these points have to do with the group leader's being effective while being both actively involved and unobtrusive–one of the crucial balancing acts to be mastered! Thus, we must guard against sins both of commission, as in the instance in which I chastened a student prematurely, and of omission, as when I left a crucial issue unaddressed. The degree of intervention can be particularly challenging in the early, formative stages of group, while safety is being assessed and developed. A great deal depends upon having created an environment in which comments can be framed and received constructively and non-defensively. In the first of these two scenarios, it was too early to be so direct. In the second, I feel in retrospect that I should have risked addressing the comment and its implications because the principle was too important and the message potentially too significant, whether it reflected addressing or ignoring the issue at hand.

This was not obvious to me at the time, however, and I have no foolproof rules or axioms to apply. It is frequently the case that there is no "right" answer, and there may not even be a "best" answer. Moreover–since we are all human and fallible–sometimes even when we are "doing our best" in any given context, it may not be "the best . . ." but simply the best we can do at that moment. Only hindsight allows me to identify how I could have improved my interaction and the potential group outcome in the scenarios I have described. We will make mistakes in our roles as group leaders, in beginnings as well as in other stages of development. The thoughtful and committed practitioner can hope, however, to make fewer and less significant mistakes over time through an ongoing process of critical self-reflection, study, seeking out coaching and training from mentor-experts and–the best teacher of all–experience.

Experience teaches, among other things, what to look for in a successful classroom group. I look for indicators such as degree of engagement in the sessions; amount of discussion and the distribution across students; respect shown for opinions of others; acquisition of course concepts and skills; demonstrated crossover between class and practice experiences; and ability to engage productively in open consideration of differences, especially around controversial topics. It is important to remember that these outcomes have their origin in strong beginnings, in seeds planted during the formation of the group.

Sometime the clearest expressions of the effectiveness of teacher group leaders come in the form of acknowledgement of the group's cohesion and productivity . . . with the facilitator featured as an invisible player. In lieu of an apple on the desk, therefore, the teacher must look for such indicators as student exclamations that, "This is the only class where we all know each others' names," or "It's great that we all feel so close and connected in this class, and are able to work and get so much done together!" The teacher-facilitator of a learning community group welcomes such comments as the planter welcomes a good harvest . . . with appreciation for the seed from which it developed, with grateful recognition of the contribution of the universe, and as evidence of a job well done.

But I Want to Do a *Real* Group:
A Personal Journey from Snubbing
to Loving to Theorizing
to Demanding Activity-Based Group Work

Whitney Wright

Flash back five years.

One morning I walked into my advisor's office with one mission: to prove my supervisor at the day treatment center was mean and stupid. I was in my first year of Social Work school, focusing on Group Work. Already, I had several years under my belt running groups with adolescents with HIV–so, I figured, I had a grasp of what a "good" group looked like. I was even starting to identify–and was haunted by–lost moments in past groups that I would meet differently this time around. Now, fueled by my new clinical training from Hunter and motivated by a placement at a psychiatric day treatment center, I was ready to start some really "therapeutic" groups. You know the kind: sex, drugs, incest, abuse, all the good stuff. The kind where the members share their most intimate secrets and emotions with the group. The kind where, as a green worker, you think that just because you're handing out tissues, you've hit the jackpot.

"My supervisor wants me to do a *sewing* group." I blurted with a sour face. "I mean, come on! That's not what Social Workers are supposed to do. I don't even know how to sew. I'm not here just to keep the mem-

[Haworth co-indexing entry note]: "But I Want to Do a *Real* Group: A Personal Journey from Snubbing to Loving to Theorizing to Demanding Activity-Based Group Work." Wright, Whitney. Co-published simultaneously in *Social Work with Groups* (The Haworth Social Work Practice Press, an imprint of The Haworth Press, Inc.) Vol. 25, No. 1/2, 2002, pp. 107-112; and: *Stories Celebrating Group Work: It's Not Always Easy to Sit on Your Mouth* (ed: Roselle Kurland, and Andrew Malekoff) The Haworth Social Work Practice Press, an imprint of The Haworth Press, Inc., 2002, pp. 107-112. Single or multiple copies of this article are available for a fee from The Haworth Document Delivery Service [1-800-HAWORTH, 9:00 a.m. - 5:00 p.m. (EST). E-mail address: getinfo@haworthpressinc.com].

107

bers busy. I'm in training to deal with the deep clinical issues my clients are experiencing. Not to make potholders. I want to do a *real* group, one about sexual decision making, or coping with mental illness, or something like that." I think I may have even whined a bit.

"Do the sewing group, Whitney," my advisor said in all-knowing tone, staring me right in the eye. "It's exactly what Social Workers are supposed to do. It'll be the best group you do all year."

Fast forward five years.

I am currently the clinical director for a program for juvenile offenders in San Francisco. Of the jobs that were offered to me when I moved here, this one paid the least, had the worst vacation and benefit package, the most unpleasant office space, and is located in a neighborhood with nary a coffee house in sight. But, unlike the others, they agreed that I could start activity-based groups with the clients and train others to join me. With many clients diagnosed with Oppositional Defiant Disorder, Conduct Disorder, Intermittent Explosive Disorder, or just filled with a lot of anger, it's only natural that impulse control and anger management are big issues. Running a boxing group that verbally addresses violence prevention while they learn a sport to be proud of and reduce their stress fits right into their world. And into my own. I've got a killer job.

The importance of activity-based group work in my practice stems from that initial sewing group. I didn't plan too much for that group–we were just going to sew, after all. I started with some fabric, needles and thread (sharpness depended on each member's dexterity), yarn, and chairs. Members worked to their own sewing skill level (a couple above that of the leader): from making a shirt or pillow, to embroidering a big knot in a piece of burlap. Then, as I sat there in the circle sewing along with the rest of the members, it was as if I was entering some parallel reality known only to those present. Unlike every other time I had shared the company of these individuals–in other groups or around the day treatment center–they seemed to be focused, awake, and actually enjoying themselves. It was as if outside this room they had been putting on a big act, a show for the tourists. Then it really happened. A few sessions in, we officially crossed over into the parallel universe. They started talking. And this was not just chitchat, and certainly not just keeping them busy. Rape, cross dressing, medication side effects, abuse, and more abuse (by family, spouse, strangers, doctors), their children taken from them, and even dreams and plans for the future when they aren't sick any more. It all came out.

Who needs Kleenex when you've got fabric?

I was awestruck. But I also knew there was something even more here. I knew that the value of using activities was not just about removing the pressure and anxiety from a face-to-face talking group by providing something to do with their hands (thus, making the talk more socially acceptable). There had to be a way to harness the group so we weren't just doing an activity and *happen* to be talking at the same time, but where the two actually jived. They needed to somehow seamlessly fit together and foster each other. I still couldn't fully answer–in a way to give justice to the richness of the experience–the questions: "Are we here to sew or to talk?" or "How is it different from a sewing class?" The endlessly offered comparison to men going fishing started becoming offensive to me. Maybe I couldn't get my head around exactly what was happening, but I could feel this was where it was at. I had converted.

So as a good grad student should, I hit the books. The literature was substantial. Activity groups had certainly been around for a while. I kept running into the adage that "social group work started with a basketball." But what did they do with that basketball and why? I found no lack of examples of benefits of activity-based group work, but no theoretical principles. And they kept calling it a "non-verbal group." What was that about? These guys were anything but non-verbal.

One afternoon, Juan, Sewer Extraordinaire, turned to me with his blue plastic needle and bright red yarn in his hand and suggested, "maybe we could make a wall hanging all together at the end." My brain synapses shot wildly. *He* knew where the group needed to go. Thanks for doing the work for me, Juan. It was a good idea. And I knew it, but I also knew there must be some distinct theoretical reason it was a good idea.

The following year I ran a two semester long co-ed ceramics group with fifteen-year-olds. The group was long enough and engaged enough for me to recognize patterns and needs of the group members as determined by the stage of group development–but fulfilled through the activity. The eternal question still vexed me: What's the purpose? Is it the process or the product or something else? It slowly unfolded: The question *is* the answer. It's all about the purpose, or shall I say purpos*es*. Clear, concise, agreed upon, and working *in tandem*.

There are two purposes in the ongoing activity group. One, mastering the activity and two, a group-wide chosen personal or community growth objective. It is this latter purpose that distinguishes the group from a class. The two need to fluctuate in their emphasis throughout the life cycle of the group. While trying to articulate the concept to a colleague, I haphazardly sketched it in graph form on a napkin (next to be published: Harry Potter and the Activity-Based Group). For us visual learners, the graph helps make tangible the theoretical framework I had been struggling with. It depicts two purposes starting separate, crossing and separating, then merging at the end. The framework eventually became an article that appeared in this journal in 1999. To illustrate the framework, I will refer to a girls' film-making group designed to help the members cope with having a parent with HIV and a boys' rock climbing group with the same personal growth purpose.

"Who are these people and can I trust them?" "What am I doing here?" "I don't know a thing about movies." To allay such unease, the activity needs to be front and center in the beginning. The role of the activity itself is to orient and unite the members and to calm some of the anxiety about the group experience and expectations regarding skill demand. The girls started out timid and guarded (mere shells of their future blunt and brazen selves). No one would even dare mention HIV. We learned about film making and script writing from a director who helped us with the technical aspects of the group. Like the members, I'd never made a movie.

Choosing a basic introductory approach to the activity–such as the boys learning basic knot tying and ballaying techniques on the climbing wall–and significant structure and assistance by the leader allows members to feel comfortable with the medium, while simultaneously encouraging commonalties to emerge. This helps the members feel accepted into the group and builds cohesiveness, vital ingredients in laying the groundwork for middles. Since they're all "in the same boat" about the activity, later we can see how deep the boat really is.

Then we get to middles. We know we're there because we can taste the spice. Members begin to know their roles in the group and they show it. The safe environment has been created and now it's time to let it all out. The activity can now take a back seat, letting the personal growth purpose cut loose. The members can choose how they want to approach the activity, acknowledging varying skill level, risk-taking, and personal differences. The individualism in the activity is mirrored in the verbal discussion. Each time we approached issues around safer sex in our script, the girls would get sidetracked and start arguing about their music taste. When called on it, they claimed they were bored. How many teens get bored while on a soap box talking about themselves? Finally, one of the girls suggested that maybe some of the members weren't using condoms paradoxically *because* of their mom's HIV status. We ended up incorporating a character into the script who puts herself at risk because she wants to be symbolically close to her mother and because she identifies so much with HIV as part of the family that getting infected seems to her an inevitable part of life.

The activity can even be put aside temporarily to focus on the discussion at hand. When we were eventually ready to roll the camera, the girls didn't want the script. Writing the script got them to a place where they didn't need it anymore. They could now sit in front of the camera with the rest of the group behind it and talk candidly about their life as a teen with an HIV-positive mom or, for a few, losing their mom to AIDS.

Meanwhile, by middles, the boys were climbing all over that wall. Though not as loquacious as the girls were, they could link conquering the high wall to other scary things in their life, like the illness or death of their parent. If they could ring that bell at the top, they could share their fear with the group.

One of the boys who wasn't as athletic as the others was having a very difficult time making it to the top. The whole group was standing with the member bellaying him. Each time he was about to ring the bell, he'd slip. The bellayer leaned back and held the rope to make sure he'd grab that wall again. They were not going to let him quit–or fall. When he finally rang the bell, sweaty with shaking legs and arms, the whole group cheared and hooted. While he was floating down sitting in his harness one of the members yelled up, "Mad up! After that, the funeral will be nothin'." A discussion of funerals the members had attended, some of them for a parent, followed. Physical and emotional trust let them physically and emotionally challenge each other. If the foundations are set in the beginning, a long and rich middle should ensue, rife with conflict, compliments, or intimate windows into members' lives never opened before. And, as group workers, the spice is scrumptious.

Let's say goodbye with a party! I don't think so. The fragile and crucial stage of endings calls for respect and planning, not just Doritos and Sprite. The activity and the existential purposes are equally emphasized. The activity needs to be conducted in a way that stimulates discussion about termination. When the girls' film was finally finished and edited, it was time for the group to come to a close. We had a screening with the group only. We talked about what is was like in the beginning and how far the group had come: now immortalized talking about sex, drugs, HIV, and Mom. They each got a copy of the film, signed by each movie star.

A group project where each member adds something helps to unite the group and allows them to experience closure together, verbally and symbolically. The boys made personal photo albums with pictures of the group and themselves on the wall and in their harnesses. We left blank pages throughout where they wrote feelings about the group and passed them around for the other members to write challenges they felt that member overcame, both physical and personal. A low minimum skill level gets them off the hook from challenging themselves as they did in middles (we wouldn't want to set them up for something they couldn't meet in the remaining time). A return to more structure provided by the group leader helps give them the stability they need as they separate from the group. The two purposes need to be discussed and evaluated by the whole group as they prepare to incorporate their group experience into their new life without it.

In retrospect, I've found that sewing or boxing or climbing or any activity–properly framed, structured, and paced–can be a powerful conduit for personal growth and clinical impact. There's not much more real than that. Yup, this is exactly what Social Workers are supposed to do.

Racial Difference and Human Commonality: The Worker-Client Relationship

Roselle Kurland

It was the Spring of 1968 and I was nearing the end of my first year of social work school at the University of Southern California. My field placement was in a community-based agency in the Watts section of Los Angeles. I worked with a group of teenage girls, all of whom were black and all of whom had been referred to the agency by the local police because they'd had a first brush with the law. I'd been working with the girls since February. Now it was May and the agency was making a panel presentation about the range of services we offered. The setting was the community room in a low-income housing project. There had been a great deal of publicity about this meeting and the room was filled.

The agency asked me to talk about the girls' group I led, to give examples of what we had been doing and discussing and to share with the audience what I saw as the ways in which the group was helpful to its members. I did that and as I sat down I was pleased and was thinking I'd done a good job of it. Other staff had spoken about other services the agency offered–a real range of kinds of services as well as of age groups reached. The presentations were followed by questions from the audience.

The first question, asked with politeness and very directly, came from a young black man: "I'd like to know how that white woman (he pointed in my direction) could possibly understand and work with black

[Haworth co-indexing entry note]: "Racial Difference and Human Commonality: The Worker-Client Relationship." Kurland, Roselle. Co-published simultaneously in *Social Work with Groups* (The Haworth Social Work Practice Press, an imprint of The Haworth Press, Inc.) Vol. 25, No. 1/2, 2002, pp. 113-118; and: *Stories Celebrating Group Work: It's Not Always Easy to Sit on Your Mouth* (ed: Roselle Kurland, and Andrew Malekoff) The Haworth Social Work Practice Press, an imprint of The Haworth Press, Inc., 2002, pp. 113-118. Single or multiple copies of this article are available for a fee from The Haworth Document Delivery Service [1-800-HAWORTH, 9:00 a.m. - 5:00 p.m. (EST). E-mail address: getinfo@haworthpressinc.com].

113

teenage girls from this community." I froze. I did not have any idea how to respond. Fortunately, the moderator of the panel, a person with a good deal of experience, answered the man's question and I did not have to. I do not remember what she said. Actually, I did not even hear her response. Nor did I hear any of the rest of the question and answer period. I remained shaken and frozen and numbed by the question. I do remember that the teenagers in my group, all of whom were present at the presentation, rushed up to me after it ended to reassure me that I was doing a great job and to express outrage at the question and at the man who asked it.

I appreciated their reassurance. But the question of what would I, as a white person, have to offer to the clients with whom I worked, many of whom would be racially different from me, stayed with me. My intent after social work school was to work with poor people in New York City. Chances are that many would be black.

Perhaps it sounds absurd that the man's question threw me to the extent that it did. But it is important to put that question in its context. That white social workers could and would be working with black clients was assumed at that time. Whether they could do so effectively was a question that simply was not asked until the 1960s and the coming of the civil rights movement. "Black power" and "black is beautiful" were ideas that had not been expressed until then.

In fact, I recall quite vividly something that had taken place only a few years before in 1965. I was working then as a newspaper reporter in Rockland County, New York and had become friendly with the black couple who headed the County's NAACP. I was at their house, sitting in the kitchen with them, when their ten-year-old son rushed in, yelling for his parents to come quickly to the living room where he was watching TV. As he saw me, though, he became embarrassed and a bit tongue-tied. What he wanted his parents to see on TV was an advertisement whose "stars" were black. That sight was so unusual at the time that it was the cause of his excitement. He was seeing black people in TV commercials for the very first time. From today's perspective, that excitement seems far away. But in 1968 the ability of white social workers to work with black clients had just not been challenged.

Following the panel presentation I went into what felt like a kind of hibernation. I thought long and hard about the question that had been addressed to me. I put myself through some intense self-examination. What *did* I have to offer, especially to black children and adolescents–the population with whom I hoped to be working–whose backgrounds were so different from my own? Could I work with them? Should I be working with them?

I'd worked before with children and adolescents who were black. But that work had been at a summer resident camp where the kids were far away from their families and their own neighborhoods. That work, I realized, had been on *my* turf rather than on theirs in the sense that it took place in a setting that *I* was familiar with, but that was new and different to the campers. Yes, at camp our aim was to create a sense of community in which the kids had as much to say as possible about what took place. But still it was different–the work took place in a well-integrated community, a kind of utopia in the outdoors where the stresses and strains and racism of the City seemed very far away. At camp, people of different races, cultures, religions, and economic strata lived together. That was what made camp, with its emphasis on the small group, so unique and so exciting. It really was utopian. But what about Watts or Harlem or Bedford-Stuyvesant or the Lower East Side? Should I be working in communities such as those where I would be the "outsider"?

The person to whom I spoke the most about my doubts was another student, a black woman from Houston, Texas, who was placed at the same agency. She was enormously helpful. She listened well. And she expressed her belief that as a white person I *could* work effectively with clients who were racially different. Given that we were working at the same agency, she knew my girls' group well. She was able to point to specific times and ways in which I had been effective in my work with them. Her specificity helped. And so did the reassurance that she offered, particularly because it came from a person who was black.

Another experience during the next year at social work school confirmed for me that as a white person I could work effectively with black clients if I were sensitive to the situations in which they were frequently placed because of their race. My field placement was at the Department of Social Services and my client, Mrs. Jones, was a black woman who was pregnant with her fourth child. Mrs. Jones was refusing to name the father of this child and would, as a result, suffer a cut in the amount of public assistance she received that would make it so low as to be impossible to live on. I, the young white worker, the ninth she had had in a period of twelve years, was the bearer of this regulation. Mrs. Jones' attitude toward me was stoic and stony. Hard as I tried, I made little progress in helping her to understand the repercussions of her decision to not reveal the father. Nor did her attitude toward me change. Our relationship remained tense, distant, and uncomfortable.

Mrs. Jones' third child, now 16 months old, had been born with severe birth defects. He had been at Childrens Hospital in Los Angeles for most of his life. Mrs. Jones lived in Pasadena and the terrible public transportation system in L.A. made it very difficult for her to visit him. She rarely saw him. One concrete way I could help Mrs. Jones was to drive her to L.A. to see her son. And so my social work role became one of chauffeur. Interestingly, the best conversations Mrs. Jones and I had took place in the car to and from Childrens Hospital.

The "breakthrough" conversation occurred following one hospital visit where I emerged feeling outraged at what had taken place. On that particular day, a change in her son's condition necessitated a number of conversations with doctors and nurses. Mrs. Jones is black, her son is black, I am white. Yet during these conversations, the medical personnel directed their words to me as if I were the child's mother and Mrs. Jones were not even present. As we were walking to the car in the parking lot afterwards, I asked Mrs. Jones, "Didn't it bother you that the doctors and nurses were talking to *me* about *your* son as if you were not even there?" It was as if I had stuck a pin in a balloon. Mrs. Jones' anger burst forth. She was, indeed, infuriated. My sensitivity to the position in which Mrs. Jones had been placed brought about a crucial turn-around in our relationship that enabled us to work together from then on.

After social work school, I did work primarily with persons of color at University Settlement House on New York City's Lower East Side. The challenge that had been presented to me at that panel in Watts and the self-examination and thinking that it precipitated served me well. I found that in my work I no longer made automatic assumptions of sameness. Yet, simultaneously, I needed to appreciate the common humanity that I shared with persons whose race and experiences were different from my own. I have come to believe that keeping in mind the balance between worker-client difference *and* commonality is essential.

Without a blatant incident such as that which took place with Mrs. Jones, however, at first in my work with persons of color I did not mention race. Looking back at it now I realize that, like the proverbial elephant in the room, race was very much there but it was something that no one, not me nor my clients, ever talked about. I was scared to talk about it directly–perhaps out of fear of being rejected, perhaps out of guilt at the benefits that I had that came about because of the white privilege that resulted from institutional racism, probably out of a mixture of both fear and guilt.

Even though race was not mentioned directly, I did feel accepted by the clients with whom I worked. I think that acceptance came about because of two qualities that were characteristic of my practice. First, I was able to communicate to clients that I genuinely cared about them. Second, I was honest with clients. I found that those qualities went a *very* long way to level the differences between us.

But differences still existed. And there was a piece of me that knew that race needed to be talked about. So hesitantly, I began to recognize out loud the racial difference between me and my clients. That did not work very well, though. My observation of racial difference brought quick and premature reassurances from clients: "Oh, that's OK," or "Don't worry about it. It's all right." But at least now I was putting racial difference out on the table so that it was no longer a taboo, no longer an area that could not be mentioned.

It took me a long time to become comfortable and adept at talking about race with clients who were different from me. I learned to not automatically raise it too early in my relationship with clients out of a sense of obligation that it "should" be raised. Instead, I found it made more sense and worked much better if I raised it because I saw some reason to do so, because I saw some way in which race might be entering into the work that was taking place.

An example is one that I use in my teaching of group work practice. It occurred in my own work with a group of single mothers. All the members of that group, as well as my co-leader, were black. I was the only white person in the room. In one meeting, the fourth of ten group sessions, the mothers were talking about situations in which they believed their children were treated unfairly by school personnel. Race was never mentioned. However, my sense was that the parents were talking about white school personnel and that they were leaving race out of their descriptions because of my presence.

When I use this example in teaching, I ask the students what they would say if they were working with this group and had the sense that race was an issue that was not being mentioned. The exact words students say they would use in bringing this to the group are not so important. What is important is that they share with the group their sense that race may be relevant to the incidents and that it may be that it is not being identified as a factor because of the presence of a white worker. What is crucial is that workers put the issue of race on the table when it arises naturally, rather than just out of a sense of obligation only.

In the actual group meeting described here, I started to share my observation about race possibly being a factor in the members' school stories. "Let me ask you a question," I said. "As the only white person in this room . . ." Before I could complete my sentence, Mrs. Thomas shouted, "Oh, we hadn't noticed . . ." Her comment brought great laughter from the group, smiles, and, I think, a sense of relief that we *all* shared. I finished my sentence by asking whether they thought race was a factor in the incidents they were describing, whether they were speaking of white school personnel treating their children unfairly. Some said they thought race was involved, others said they did not. The important message to the group, though, was that race could be talked about here. Also, my comment demonstrated that societal racism could have an impact upon the group members, that it needed to be taken into account in discussion of their experiences.

The commonalities shared by the members of this group, as relatively isolated and struggling single parents, caused them to bond quickly. Each week at the end of the meeting the group members would stand and chat for at least a half hour at the coat rack outside the meeting room. Goodbyes were said with warm hugs among them. It is interesting that after the meeting described here the members included me in their goodbye rituals. Up until then I had not been included. Now for the first time, the group members hugged me too.

Addressing race with clients whose race is different from my own has been a progression for me: from thinking it did not matter, to wondering whether it did, to knowing that it did but being fearful of talking about it, to talking about it immediately and prematurely, to becoming comfortable enough to wait to raise it until it comes up in a way that flows naturally in the work with clients.

In addition, I have learned to look not just at racial difference between me and the clients with whom I work. I need to look beyond the personal and to view the social meanings that race has, to take those meanings into account and to help clients to do so rather than unfairly assign blame to themselves personally when what is taking place is societally motivated. Above all, I have learned that racial difference can be talked about. It needs to be.

Hidden Treasure Under the Rabi Tree:
A Group Worker's Journey
from Haiti to the US

Roseline Felix

I once read a book called *The Butterfly's Way*, about the Haitian's Dyaspora in the United States. In the introduction there is a statement by Jean-Claude Martineau, who refers to the Haitian culture. He says, "If you don't know the butterfly's way, you will pass it by without noticing: it's so well hidden in the grass."

I see group work in a similar way, as a hidden treasure. If one is unfamiliar with the concept of group culture, which can be discovered throughout the group process, one can miss out on the wonders that lay beneath, the hidden treasure. With this in mind, I will share my early observations and experiences of the power of groups. These experiences have helped me to understand that individuals can achieve their needs and goals when they work together.

GROWING UP IN HAITI

Thinking about writing this article brought me back to the days when I was eleven or twelve years old in Dondon, Haiti. Reflecting back, I began to understand how the Rabi (pronounced RAH-bee) tree, located in

[Haworth co-indexing entry note]: "Hidden Treasure Under the Rabi Tree: A Group Worker's Journey from Haiti to the US." Felix, Roseline. Co-published simultaneously in *Social Work with Groups* (The Haworth Social Work Practice Press, an imprint of The Haworth Press, Inc.) Vol. 25, No. 1/2, 2002, pp. 119-128; and: *Stories Celebrating Group Work: It's Not Always Easy to Sit on Your Mouth* (ed: Roselle Kurland, and Andrew Malekoff) The Haworth Social Work Practice Press, an imprint of The Haworth Press, Inc., 2002, pp. 119-128. Single or multiple copies of this article are available for a fee from The Haworth Document Delivery Service [1-800-HAWORTH, 9:00 a.m. - 5:00 p.m. (EST). E-mail address: getinfo@haworthpressinc.com].

119

front of my house, acted as a vehicle for group interaction and how it would later contribute to inspire me to become a group worker.

As I am writing, I can visualize myself sitting on the stoop of my house facing the Rabi tree. This enormous structure, with its outreaching branches and leaves–like a huge umbrella–served as a meeting place under which people from the community gathered. Beneath its soothing, refreshing shade people socialized. For example, merchants sold their wares, neighbors played dominoes, and children chased one another and played soccer.

Across the street was the Catholic Church where parishioners attended mass and other church activities. To the left of the church was the parochial school for boys, with its rectory. To the right of the church were the theater, some private houses, and an old police precinct. Behind the church was a girls' parochial school, a community clinic, and a cemetery. On school days during lunchtime students sat under the tree to study, help others with their homework, or just hang out with friends. On weekends or holidays, groups gathered and had bicycle races, played volleyball, basketball, or football. At other times, under the shade and coolness of the Rabi tree, different groups gathered to play cards, dominoes, plan trips or other activities, and discuss a variety of community issues. Occasionally, there were heated discussions that lead to fights. Eventually all conflicts were amicably resolved within the informal group.

In addition to the economic benefits derived for those who sold their wares, the social interactions under the Rabi tree created a sense of belonging that resulted in many friendships and a growing network of support and resources that was consistently available and essential for the survival of the people living in the community.

AN EARLY LESSON IN MUTUAL AID, UNDER THE RABI TREE

I recall a profound experience that made me acutely aware of how group interaction and collective effort can make a difference. It was a Saturday, about midday, when I saw this couple sitting under the Rabi tree. The lady was pregnant and about to give birth. She was experiencing great pain. However, the local clinic was closed. She had no place to go. Several passers-by came and offered her support in an effort to comfort her. They held her hand, offered cool water, and spoke soothingly. One of the good Samaritans knew that my uncle, a physician, was in town on vacation. She called him for help.

My uncle examined the pregnant lady and determined that she was experiencing complications and had to be driven to the hospital in the next town. Immediately! Experiencing this mutual effort first hand, a collective will to assist someone in time of need became a driving force and inspiration for me throughout my life. I realized that if these caring neighbors did not put aside their needs to help this lady, both mother and child could have died.

These early observations under the Rabi tree have made me aware that everyone has something to offer, provided that they are willing to work together to help one another. However, I came to realize that no matter how good the intentions, the attainment of mutual goals will sometimes be served best under the umbrella and supervision of skilled and professional guidance. This is something that led me to social work and, ultimately, group work.

BEYOND THE RABI TREE

Other significant encounters that have guided me towards group work include witnessing social, political and economic injustice. For example, seeing a talented child being deprived of an education because of his lower social status and lack of finances; painfully observing women, with little or no resources, lacking a political voice; and seeing their "macho" men denied the opportunity to actualize themselves, becoming background shadows in their families. The pain that this has evoked in me is the impetus that has driven me to become an audible voice, a moving force–an advocate.

Becoming a group worker has changed my perception of how I see individuals both personally and professionally. I have come to realize that in a group each individual is like a unique piece of a puzzle that, when combined with others, creates a powerful force of talents and ideas. I have come to appreciate how, through cooperative exchange, a group can influence change in social, economic and political spheres. Through group work I have become acutely aware of how a society is dependent upon the collective efforts of its individual members to survive, each individual being a significant part of a greater whole.

As a first generation Haitian-American who knows the spiritual nature and cultural values of the Haitian community, I chose to become a social worker with the idea of working with other Haitian-American immigrants. I thought that maybe I could re-create the spirit of the Rabi tree by using my newly developing knowledge and skills as a group worker. Working at North Shore Child and Family Guidance Center, a children's mental health center in Long Island, New York, gave me the opportunity to do just that, to begin to create what has become known as the Haitian Family Life Program. But I knew that I couldn't do it alone.

"DO YOU SPEAK CREOLE?"

"Do you speak Creole?" asked eight year old Monique as she gazed into my eyes searching for a connection. She waited patiently for a reply. To this day I remember the radiance of her smiling face when I answered, "Yes."

Monique held my hand and proceeded to walk beside me down the hallway. When we arrived at my office I explained my role in the school. Her ears seemed to perk up when I mentioned the part about helping students born in Haiti adapt to their new country. She expressed feelings about her struggle and confusion living in the US with its different customs and values. Especially frustrating was the task of learning a new language. I told her that the purpose of the group I was forming was to help the members to do better in school, academically and socially.

After meeting with all of the referred students I made contact with their parents who described similar struggles with their adopted home. It soon became clear that my work in the group with the children would just be part of my role. I decided to form a parallel group for parents to become more aware of community resources and more adept at accessing them. I thought that a good first step would be to establish trust with the parents and their children. This could be a stepping stone to a mediating process between home and school that would reduce the widening gap in understanding and improve cooperation.

RESURRECTING THE SPIRIT OF THE RABI TREE

I discovered that the road to the parents was through an influential clergyman in town, a reverend who I had come to know. He was excited about my work and plans and introduced me to the congregation. He offered the church as a meeting place.

The Haitian Family Life Program (HFLP), a cluster of services for parents and their children, gradually grew from an initial series of bi-weekly meetings which were held Sunday afternoons at All Saints

Church. Its leader, Rev. Wilbert Dorilus, is a well known leader within the Haitian community in Westbury/New Cassel, Long Island, New York. He played a major role in providing his facility as a meeting place and encouraged parents to learn about the American system. Parents trusted him because of his fine reputation and role as church leader. Thus, he facilitated their attendance on Sunday afternoons and encouraged free expression. They felt safe in this place. I knew I couldn't create a program without the support of Reverend Wilbert.

Meetings at All Saints Church provided new immigrants with the opportunity to come together in a trusting environment, a safe place where they shared concerns and learned about their new community. The gatherings helped members to deal with feelings of isolation and helplessness, limitations due to language barriers, and unfamiliarity with the American system. It made them aware of services and resources available to them. As they continued to attend meetings, members slowly earned each other's trust.

The issue of trust has always been crucial for Haitians. This is due to a long history of living under oppressive governments, colonization, and dictatorships. Since I am from Haiti, I am acutely aware of the psychological and social impact these fear-producing governing systems can create. Having had similar life experiences enables me to effectively plan strategies to reach out to this community. For example, knowing the significant impact that the Haitian church has always had among my people, I decided that working together with a church leader in a church setting was the most effective way to make connections. Within a safe environment, participants were able to openly present problems, exchange ideas, and discuss relevant issues. As a result, an effective program designed to address their needs took root–the birth of a new Rabi tree.

The following year, in addition to the bi-weekly meetings at the church, a series of parent workshops were offered along with an English class. The purpose of the English class/workshop was to teach parents English and to raise awareness about different resources. Guest speakers such as lawyers, health care professionals, educators, and others were invited to share their knowledge. I think that if my uncle (the doctor) was nearby he would have rolled up his sleeves and pitched in, just like he did that day under the Rabi tree in Dondon. The presentations helped to demystify the educational system (and other systems). They had the effect of reviving the parents who seemed out of breath trying to figure everything out, not clearly understanding their rights. In addition to helping them learn English, this program also helped them gain parenting skills and, most significantly, helped them build trust and mutual support.

REACHING BACK TO THINK AHEAD AND BUILD TRUST

As the group evolved, I started to observe certain behaviors among group members, which caused me to reflect back to my own early experiences in the United States. One evening, I observed how individuals separated themselves into informal subgroups composed of those who knew some English and those who did not. Each group isolated themselves from the other. I knew right away how some of them felt. I remembered my first few weeks in an ESL (English as a Second Language) class and how isolated I felt. I was very intimidated and felt at a loss. Not knowing the language accentuated how different I felt. It wasn't a nice feeling at all. Since I did not know the students, I was unsure about how they felt about me. At times, some of them tried to show off their language skills by asking the teacher questions to subjects that they already knew. I appreciated how the teacher did her best to make me feel comfortable, by having someone translate what she was teaching. Having had these experiences sensitized me to the needs of the parents' group. Therefore, I was able to reach out and bridge the gap between the advanced and less advanced.

I also became aware of how important it is for a group worker to effectively intervene when a disruptive force or obstacle has a negative affect on achieving the group's purpose. For example, in one learning group, several mothers brought their children to class. As one would expect, they behaved as children. They were boisterous in their play, jumped out of their seats, some argued, and so forth. Needless to say, the members of the class could not concentrate. Although quite annoyed, not wanting to offend their classmates, they stoically bore these disruptive intrusions. Realizing that their non-challenging response could be culturally related, I intervened. Aware of their respect for authority, I directly encouraged them to express their feelings and explore ways in which the children could be managed, at the same time learning could be facilitated.

The parents were very responsive. For example, it was suggested that some parents could sit with the children while others were learning. Others discussed the possibility of leaving the children with responsible babysitters. This conversation raised the issue of how they would have handled this matter if they were back home. They talked about extended family members and friends that they could leave their children with. They reflected on how life was drastically different in the United States.

Most immigrants struggle with the norms of both worlds as they attempt to adjust and embrace their new environment. For this reason, a worker must be aware of these cultural conflicts and address them as they surface. It is also important for immigrants to become aware of information and resources to help them navigate and adjust to their new culture.

Similar to the holding environment and the safety that the Rabi tree provided by its shade and cool breeze, a group leader must promote an enlightened atmosphere in which the group can be nurtured; a place where people can securely relax as they get their needs met and where members can feel comfortable enough to work out their concerns and learn from one another. In other words, a place of trust.

I identified with several experiences that some of the individuals shared in the parent class. When I arrived here, I did not know my way around. I did not trust myself to go out. I was afraid that I could get lost and not be able to find my way back. I was not clear about the laws of this country. I had only the knowledge that I brought with me. I had to depend on someone else for basic instructions. For example, a classmate walked me to the school cafeteria and accompanied me to my classroom at the end of recess.

In one of the group discussions regarding how to get around town, a parent shared similar feelings. Marie wanted to find out how she could get to a place where she was told that she could find a job. She further explained that she had been in the country for a year and didn't know how to take the bus. She was concerned that she would miss the interview and never get the job because she did not know her way around. Another member, Louis, asked her if she knew the address. Marie then stated the address. It happened that Louis worked in that town. He offered her a ride and then both exchanged phone numbers. Other members were very helpful in giving her information about different bus stops and identified different bus numbers that pass through the town. Marie was successful in using resources outside and inside the group to help her to find a job.

As new arrivals came to town from Haiti, word about the group spread. The newcomers requested to have similar meetings available to them.

The group has allowed the parents to have the opportunity to share common experiences in a trusting atmosphere. They asked to have this type of program continue on an ongoing basis. At the members' request, the group continued in order to help the members develop communication skills and competence around issues of daily life. The group program expanded to include local trips, parent conferences, practice at completing job application forms, and learning advocacy skills.

The information, interaction, and feedback helped the parents to become empowered. With opportunities to go on trips, practice language skills, and network with others, parents became more involved in their children's academic lives. Many have attended meetings in school that they would have previously avoided, and shared information they have received with others in their group.

A PAUSE FOR CELEBRATION, APPRECIATION, AND RECOGNITION

At the end of the most recent school year, the parents decided to hold an evening of recognition and cultural awareness. The goal was to thank agency and school personnel and others who lent support in putting the program together. The event was held in the local elementary school where the parents attended a weekly ESL/Parenting workshop series.

Brief speeches of thanks were made in the auditorium. Certificates of completion and appreciation were awarded to parents and workshop providers. Local media covered the event and took photographs of the proud parents as their children and other relatives and friends looked on and applauded. A moving show of Haitian painting, sculpture, and folk art was displayed. This was accompanied by traditional music and a delicious Haitian meal including Haitian pastry, rice with black mushrooms, pumpkin soup, and conchs, among other delights. No one went away hungry.

The cultural awareness and recognition night was a good example of a group using its internal and external resources to reach a goal on the way to social change. Everyone involved worked cooperatively to make the celebration enjoyable. A new ritual, what was to become an annual event, was created. It felt just like the type of collective effort that I observed and experienced under the Rabi tree.

CONCLUSION

My childhood memories and my group work experiences have allowed me to be more conscious of my surroundings and the need to tap resources within and outside of the group. When working with a group, I am often reminded of the hidden treasures I discovered under the protective shade of the Rabi tree. I always keep in mind that each individual has a talent which will surface at some point during the life of the group. The individual talents, when nurtured and developed, can be utilized collectively to strengthen the group and help members to move forward. Helping members to discover, tap, and share resources, the treasures within themselves and in their environments, can give them strength and improve the quality of their lives.

REFERENCE

Danticat, Edwidge. (2001). *The Butterfly's Way: Voices from the Haitian Dyaspora in the United States.* New York: Soho Press, Inc. New York.

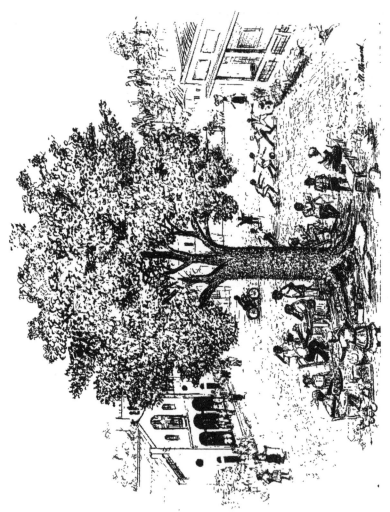

The word "Rabi tree" is a popular name that people use in Dondon Haiti for the Hura crepitans, a tree that contains spines around its stem and branches. This plant belongs to the Euphorbiaceae family. It is also known as Sablier in Haiti, Javillo in Santo-Domingo, and Sand-Box tree in Jamaica. © Apollon Menard. Used with permission.

Navigating in Groups . . .
Experiencing the Cultural as Political

Flavio Francisco Marsiglia

In this article, I reflect upon my shared experiences of practicing social work with groups in a variety of settings during the past two decades.
During that time I have come to conceptualize group membership as vessels at sea. During the pre-group phase members are navigating on their
own until the group worker, serving as the initial caller, loosely brings
them together. Once the vessels (members) agree on a common direction (purpose) and a set of navigation rules, they start to develop a sense
of belonging (identity) as they navigate toward the agreed upon direction. In due time, the individual vessels grow into a strong flotilla (the
group). The power of the group becomes a shared compass that allows
them to sail through challenging and tempestuous waters into the safety
of new harbors (termination phase). After resting and celebrating, vessels depart on their own to explore new worlds and in some cases to as-
semble new flotillas. It is through this maritime metaphor that I will
provide an overview of my group experiences with diverse populations.

Social workers are often summoned to facilitate these gatherings of
diverse vessels, at unfamiliar shores, adventuring into unknown seas. It
is at those times that the most beautiful discoveries take place, when our
sense of direction becomes challenged, and when new compasses are
invented. Facilitating diverse groups at unique environments has provided me with invaluable opportunities to enter extraordinary worlds.
My formal social work education provided me with an essential knowl-

[Haworth co-indexing entry note]: "Navigating in Groups . . . Experiencing the Cultural as Political."
Marsiglia, Flavio Francisco. Co-published simultaneously in *Social Work with Groups* (The Haworth Social
Work Practice Press, an imprint of The Haworth Press, Inc.) Vol. 25, No. 1/2, 2002, pp. 129-137; and: *Stories
Celebrating Group Work: It's Not Always Easy to Sit on Your Mouth* (ed: Roselle Kurland, and Andrew
Malekoff) The Haworth Social Work Practice Press, an imprint of The Haworth Press, Inc., 2002, pp. 129-137.
Single or multiple copies of this article are available for a fee from The Haworth Document Delivery Service
[1-800-HAWORTH, 9:00 a.m. - 5:00 p.m. (EST). E-mail address: getinfo@haworthpressinc.com]

129

edge-base of working with groups. It was through the doing, however, that the accumulated knowledge came alive, was tested, reformulated, and enhanced. Different world views emerged through the group experiences. For the purpose of this article, I have elected to describe some of those experiences where the cultural became political (Sanchez and Pita, 1999). The cultural competency ideal often became challenged by the political undercurrents affecting the groups (Renshon and Duckitt, 1997). The following group narratives illustrate this phenomenon.

SOCIAL WORK INTERNS TRANSPORTED BACK–IN GROUP– TO THE SPANISH CIVIL WAR

My initiation into the cultural as political dimension of group work took place during my group work field practicum. I was assigned to a continued care facility for the elderly sponsored by the Spanish embassy in Montevideo, Uruguay. A large percentage of the residents had emigrated to their new country during or immediately after the Spanish Civil War (Persing, 1999). My classmates and I were instructed by our field supervisor to be aware of infusing appropriate cultural content into our groups. Culture for us meant a generic "Spanish" culture. As we began our work, we were challenged and educated by the experience.

One of the group members, a distinguished looking gentleman in his late 70s, whom I will call Don Esteban, was very active in group. Suddenly he stopped attending the weekly sessions. We were informed that he was ill and that the doctor had prescribed him to rest. Group members decided on different roles they were willing to take during his convalescence and agreed to keep him informed about group activities.

One morning as we arrived to the residence, the receptionist gave us a note from Don Esteban. He was asking us to inform the priest about his illness and his desire to receive daily communion in his room. We found the note peculiar. Why was he asking us to deliver such a message? He knew that half of the interns were Jewish, while most of the residents were Catholic. More importantly, we, the interns, did not live there.

We raised the issue in group. Members were unusually quiet. Finally, after much prompting, Doña Dolores explained that Don Esteban had already asked her for the same favor. She consulted with the group and they agreed not to inform the priest about his request because Don Esteban was a "socialist." Suddenly, members became very engaged in a passionate debate. Thousands of miles away from Spain, and several decades later, it felt as if the Spanish Civil War had not yet ended.

Suddenly, we–a group of young social work interns–were involved in a religious and political dilemma for which we felt completely unprepared. It took the group several sessions and the return of Don Esteban to adequately process the incident. We had to take a back seat approach and listen to the stories. Some members were losing their short term memory, but during those sessions they were able to describe in great detail their Civil War experiences. The group decided that their behavior was inappropriate and one by one they apologized to Don Esteban.

After the conflict, the group became stronger and members became active in different activities, promoting a better understanding between members of the two opposite factions in the old war. Doña Dolores and Don Esteban became co-chairs of the reconciliation committee.

The described residential setting was a microcosm of the stories of the residents. Distance and exile kept the residents away from the national healing that was taking place in Spain. The group became the forum where the ghosts of the past were confronted, a past that was very much present in the daily life of the residents. To be Spanish was not enough. They needed other adjectives such as *falangista, republicano,* or *socialista* to truly describe their identities. The cultural and the political were one and the same. The "communion conflict" helped the members advance to the next stage of group development. The incident gave me a new appreciation for the confluence of the political and the cultural. It also prepared me for future experiences as I navigated through other seas and encountered unexpected shores.

A "CITY BOY" FACILITATING GROUPS WITH RURAL YOUTH

One such journey took place as I was working at a youth agency where I was helping form and facilitate youth groups in the countryside of Uruguay. I was born and raised in the city. My previous ventures into the countryside (or as city residents call it, the *interior*) were related to camping trips with the Boy Scouts or family vacations. I did not know the culture of the *interior* and I was a bit self-conscious about my "city boy" outlook.

Most of my work took place during weekends. Small town parishes served as my conduit to young people. I would often spend the night at parish houses or at group members' homes. In most areas I went there were no hotels and in towns big enough for hotels, my contacts would have been offended if I even had suggested checking-in at the local hotel.

Traditional gaucho barbecues, guitar playing, and singing were always part of the group meetings. Many of my book-learned concepts about group work needed some adaptation to be applicable in those times and in that environment. For example, one of the youth groups used to meet at a remote chapel in the middle of the pampas (hilly grasslands). Starting time was approximate, as they waited for the last member to arrive before beginning the sessions. Usually I was the first one to arrive. I had been instructed by the group to boil water, prepare, and later serve *maté* (a ritualistic South American tea).

A strong code of hospitality was observed. Protecting one's boundaries in a clinical sense would have been plain rude. Taking care of each other meant much more than active listening. The country was going through rough times, the political waters were stormy, anti-democratic winds were targeting the very soul of the nation. Groups were a refuge, a risky act of defiance, and a tool for change.

Much of group work in those days was based on the consciousness raising writings of the Brazilian philosopher Paulo Freire (1985). Freire had the distinction of being among a long list of authors banned by the governing dictatorship, 1973-1984 (Roniger, Sznajder, and Skaar, 2001). Censorship became real as I became involved with several groups located in an area bordering Brazil. This particular set of groups organized a gathering to share their experiences, applying "praxis," and to receive additional training on Freire's method. The regional army chief learned about the gathering and forbade holding the session. Young people had traveled from distant points in the region and were not willing to go back home without achieving the stated purpose for the meeting.

A principal of a small school on the other side of the international border learned over the radio about the ban and offered her school building on the Brazilian side as an alternative meeting place. Unanimously, the youth accepted the invitation and decided–in protest–to march across the border. After a long hour walk under the midday sun, the youth arrived safely to the school cafeteria where a delicious traditional meal (*fresuada*) awaited them.

This example illustrates how the political, geographic, and cultural context influenced the life of the groups. During the described unfortunate political era, groups were often the only tools available to maintain civil society alive. Food, shelter, and other expressions of hospitality were an intrinsical part of the group process. The context, however, transformed traditionally cultural ritual into political gestures of defiance. Each group decision and group action kept alive the flame of a long democratic tradition that the regime was attempting to extinguish.

Groups were harbors of dignity in a very undignified sea. Some young women and men involved in such groups were eventually arrested, others had no other alternative than to go into exile. Despite all the repression, the spirit of democracy was kept alive and eventually the regime collapsed under the weight of its own anachronism.

FACILITATING AN ARAB YOUNG WOMEN'S ISSUES GROUP

The early 1990s found me in Cleveland, working as a bilingual school social worker. I was assigned to develop and facilitate a drop out prevention program for limited English proficient middle school students. I had the joy of working with children and families of many cultural backgrounds. There were many student groups. One group that taught me unique lessons was the Arabic young women's group. The school district became aware of an unusually high drop out rate among young Arabic-speaking female students. These girls were high achievers and attended school regularly; however, as they got older many of them were dropping-out and not enrolling in high school. As we investigated the trend, we learned that the majority of these Arabic speaking students were Palestinian refugees and immigrants.

We formed a group with the purpose of discussing the female student's school experiences. I recruited an Arabic speaking acquaintance to be my volunteer co-facilitator; I will call her Fatima. It took a few weeks to get all the consent forms signed by the parents. Fatima helped me conduct home visits to explain the purpose of the group to a few doubtful parents.

Soon after the group started to meet, we learned that some of the students were preparing to participate in their pre-arranged weddings. They needed to go back to their village or refugee camp of origin to participate in the ceremony and it was understood that upon their return they were not going back to school. Some of the remaining Lebanese, Syrian, and other Palestinian students (Moslem and Christian) were very vocal in their disapproval of the practice. My initial reaction to the stories was one of puzzlement and helplessness. Fatima took the driver's seat. She asked me and the other group members who presented themselves as "urban" to avoid giving speeches and to listen to the girls. As we became better listeners, we began to understand the difficult balancing act these girls were performing.

They were expressing their desire to continue with their education and at the same time they wanted to follow the traditional ways. Fatima taught us not to put down the culture and the family while we helped look for alternatives. Some parents became concerned with their daughters' participation in the group. My inability to speak Arabic made me completely dependent on Fatima. In group we searched for alternatives. The group members became supportive of each other instead of just critical of each other.

Negotiating within the culture was proven to be the most effective tool. Some weddings were delayed, others took place as planned but the new husbands and the brides' parents were visited by group members. A wedding fund was established and gifts were bought and presented by the group members. Those visits served as a bridge between the families' culture and the school's culture. Some of the original group members in time became younger "Fatimas," bi-cultural women able to navigate through two different worlds and able to reconcile apparently unreconcilable dreams.

The Arabic-speaking young women's group took me to shores I have never seen before. My lack of experience with the culture made me vulnerable. My own vulnerability made me grow and learn. The experience challenged many of my most basic beliefs and attitudes about education, women's rights, and cultural traditions. The safety of the group and Fatima's presence neutralized some of my ethnocentric attitudes and practices. As I look back to that experience, I wonder about the generosity and hospitality I experienced in group and at many of the girls' homes.

CREATING VIDEOS IN GROUP
WITH MEXICAN AMERICAN ADOLESCENTS

My concluding story took place in the late 1990s in Phoenix. At that time I was wearing the researcher hat. The National Institutes of Health/National Institute on Drug Abuse funded a study to develop and test a culturally-grounded approach to drug prevention among pre-adolescents in the Southwest. At the core of the effort was the development of educational videos by high school students to be used to teach middle school students prevention messages. The videos were based on narratives we collected from middle school students about ways in which they resisted drugs. We gave the narratives to the high school students and asked them to develop scripts, audition for the characters and produce the videos for us. The student producers were enrolled in the media program and had the expertise needed to conduct the "mission."

The premise behind this effort was to have kids producing prevention messages for kids. Again, we used Paulo Freire's teaching to guide us in using "praxis" as a method for group process and outcomes (Freire, 1995). I worked more closely with one of the student groups. Mexican Americans constituted the numerical majority of this group. The group members had known each other for years. Most of them were neighbors, classmates, and in some cases relatives and friends. The group went through the pre-group phase very quickly. The group purpose was two-fold: Students aimed to increase their awareness about ethnic identity and drug use and at the same time produce a set of educational videos for the prevention curriculum.

The charge to the group was to be "in charge." Social workers and teachers involved in the project conveyed the message that the group had the power to produce the videos they wanted from the script to the final editing. Adults were there to provide support, not to lead the process. To evaluate the process we use a technique called "video ethnography" (Wasson, 2000). A university graduate student video-taped the student group sessions. After a month of filming videotapes, we reviewed the videos with the students and evaluated the group process. Some interesting themes emerged.

For example, although they were formally in control, they were not exercising it. The video ethnography showed how they were looking for answers from the adults and were having a hard time exercising their autonomy. It was very difficult for the students to embrace the new approach to creativity and power within the pre-established structure of the school. The content of the scripts came across as moralistic and stereotypical. The youth were repeating the standard messages young people receive from adults. Although the ethnographic data was telling them that most teens do not use drugs, they were emphasizing drug use versus drug resistance. Stereotypes about teens and about Mexican Americans emerged and were questioned and changed. Using "praxis," students became aware of these shortcomings and over time they overcame them. In group they rehearsed new behaviors that allowed them to gain control over the process of producing the educational videos.

In time, students developed the scripts, conducted auditions, and successfully filmed and edited the videos. The product of their work became the centerpiece of an innovative prevention curriculum that was tested with approximately 6,000 students. The videos were recognized by the film community through Emmy and International Videos Awards.

We learned many lessons from the experience. For example, we understood more clearly the powerful influence that social context has on groups (Hays and Ellickson, 1996). The group members were young and Mexican American, two identities that have excluded them from true participation in certain settings. The project asked them to be at the center of the creative process, to take the lead, to make decisions, and to have a voice. But just by giving them such a charge, we could have not expected an immediate response. There was a need to develop trust.

The video ethnography served as a mirror for the group members and the group facilitators. The members were not claiming the new waters and the adults were not sharing their turf. The cultural became political as students were afraid of using Spanish terms or traditional Mexican symbols as part of the video scenarios. Previous rejections made them protective of their culture. As part of an internally colonized minority (Blauner, 1972) they were reticent to share cultural products and to be themselves. It took time and trust building to engender in the students a sense that this group was different. The group facilitators also had to prove themselves in order for the young men and women to feel safe enough to raise their anchor and sail through their creative journey.

DISCUSSION

The four group experiences presented in this article took place in different contexts but shared a common journey through the waters of culture and politics. They took us across imaginary and real boundaries, exposing us to different shores but similar journeys. These groups–as all groups–are microcosms of larger societies. The described groups were not floating in the air; they were navigating on real waters moved by unique cultural and political currents. The groups became stronger as they learned how to recognize and embrace those currents. Quiet waters often do not allow for real groups to emerge. Our role is often to encourage and support the vessels to venture into the open sea. The image of the open sea brings to mind a liberal English translation of the ancient motto of the city of Paris: *To navigate is essential; to linger is not essential.*

REFERENCES

Blauner, R. (1972). *Racial Oppression in America.* New York: Harper & Row.
Freire, P. (1995). *Pedagogy of the Oppressed.* New York: Continuum.
Hays, R. D. and Ellickson, P.L. (1996). What is adolescent alcohol misuse in the United States according to the experts? *Alcohol and Alcoholism, 31,* 3, 297-303.

Persing, B. (1999). Arms for Spain: The untold story of the Spanish Civil War. *Library Journal, 124,* 14, 210-221.

Renshon, S. and Duckitt, J. (1997). Cultural and cross-cultural political psychology: Toward the development of a new subfield. *Political Psychology, 18,* 2, 233-240.

Roniger, L., Sznajder, M., and Skaar, E. (2001). The legacy of human rights violations in the Southern Cone: Argentina, Chile, and Uruguay. *Latin American Politics and Society, 43,* 1, 149-153.

Sanchez R. and Pita, B. (1999). Mapping cultural/political debates in Latin American studies. *Cultural Studies, 13,* 2, 290-318.

Wasson, C. (2000). Ethnography in the field of design. *Human Organization, 59,* 4, 377-388.

Learning to Talk About Taboo Subjects:
A Lifelong Professional Challenge

Lawrence Shulman

Every society and social group develops a culture. The culture includes, among other things, norms of behavior, values, roles for its members, rules of interaction, and a usually informal list of taboo subjects. For some groups, the list can be formalized. When we work with more than one person at a time we create an "entity" that is more than the sum of its parts. It is this group culture that defines this entity, which I refer to as the group-as-a-whole (Shulman, 1999). While we can't see this entity, we infer its existence through the behaviors of the group members. If everyone acts as if a norm of behavior is held in common, and an unspoken agreement has been reached to avoid a taboo area, then we can infer that this is a property of the group's culture and that members feel they must respect it.

A major problem for the group worker is that the group's culture can be one that either encourages effective work (a culture for work) or blocks effective work. A second major problem for the group worker is that she or he has more than likely been exposed to the very same culture as the members, shares their norms and is just as reluctant to enter a taboo area. This leads to the problem referred to by William Schwartz as the "illusion of work" (Schwartz, 1961). I have thought of it as a kind of dance, a "pas des deux," in which the group members and the leader carry on a conversation while nothing real is happening. It's as if all are respecting an invisible sign on the wall that says: *In this group, we will*

[Haworth co-indexing entry note]: "Learning to Talk About Taboo Subjects: A Lifelong Professional Challenge." Shulman, Lawrence. Co-published simultaneously in *Social Work with Groups* (The Haworth Social Work Practice Press, an imprint of The Haworth Press, Inc.) Vol. 25, No. 1/2, 2002. pp. 139-150; and: *Stories Celebrating Group Work: It's Not Always Easy to Sit on Your Mouth* (ed: Roselle Kurland, and Andrew Malekoff) The Haworth Social Work Practice Press, an imprint of The Haworth Press, Inc., 2002, pp. 139-150. Single or multiple copies of this article are available for a fee from The Haworth Document Delivery Service [1-800-HAWORTH, 9:00 a.m. - 5:00 p.m. (EST). E-mail address: getinfo@haworthpressinc.com].

not discuss sex, race, sexual orientation, death, abuse, rage, religion, class, shame, guilt, mental illness, disability, substance abuse, fears of all kinds, angry reactions to the worker or other members, or any other subjects that would simultaneously make the work of the group real but also painful and frightening for the members and the leader(s). Violation of these rules may result in social isolation or even exclusion from the group.

Because I have always viewed the group using an "organismic" model (the group as an organism), rather than a "mechanistic" model (the group as a machine), I have been able to see growth and change over time resulting from internal interactions among members and the leader and external interactions with the environment. The group members (and even the leader) usually immediately establish the larger societal culture in the group. However, the culture can change, evolve and strengthen to be able to address even the most difficult taboo subjects. In fact, this is one of the most essential tasks of the group leader. The leader must help the group members identify the existence of the culture, taboos and all, and then challenge them in order to change the culture. To implement this role, group leaders must first look inward and confront their personal and professional fears in order to develop the skill and courage to help others do the same.

The balance of this article is my recollection of my own forty-year professional and personal journey in learning to deal with taboo subjects. It is illustrated with a number of examples: some embarrassing examples of how I avoided issues; others in which I caught my mistakes almost as I made them; still others that I look back upon with professional pride. It also illustrates that the process never stops and that we continue to grow professionally by continually examining our work. Failing to do this, we start to decline and lose whatever skills and understanding we have developed. There is no such thing as professionally "standing still."

THE EARLY YEARS:
WHAT I DID AND DIDN'T LEARN
IN MY MSW TRAINING

I was a group work major in my MSW program at a time (1959 to 1961) when the practice settings and the literature were based upon years of work in community centers, settlement houses, local and national youth service programs, educational settings, etc. Social group work as a modality of practice for addressing personal and social problems, such as life threatening illnesses, psychiatric illness, substance abuse and recovery, had not yet fully developed. Of the 30 group workers in my graduating class, 29 went to work in the community settings described above, and only one joined a social work department in a psychiatric hospital. For many of us, our first positions as proud MSWs were as supervisors of programs employing untrained group leaders.

Given this context, it was not surprising that much of our attention to "method," what we actually did with groups, focussed on the use of program activities such as singing, games, dancing, films, etc. We were the envy of our casework major peers at school as they passed the open door of our "activity" class and saw us having such a good time. (They were also not overly focussed on method because of the existing professional educational paradigm that emphasized assessment and diagnosis, but was short on issues of intervention.) If group workers identified a problem in a group, such as scapegoating, we would try to solve it by indirect means such as suggesting activities at which the scapegoat could excel. We would rarely address the process directly and had little understanding that the dynamics were actually the group members' means of raising their own taboo concerns (e.g., fear of masculine identity expressed by adolescent boys who scapegoated the weakest and smallest group member). It was only after graduation, and as I began to more intensively examine my work and the practice of students that I supervised, that I began to both understand the meaning of the process and to develop effective interventions to address the issues directly. I first had to understand my own reluctance to open such a discussion, my fear of hurting the scapegoat, and my identification with the scapegoat, having had a similar experience as a youth myself.

Given the social context within which my education took place, it is no surprise that I did get a wonderful introduction to issues of social justice and civil rights. I had early mentors in both class and field who went on to be national social work leaders and advocates for a social work professional role that addressed what Schwartz, quoting C. Wright Mills, described as a concern for both "private troubles" and "public issues" (Schwartz, 1969). However, because of the lack of understanding and attention to method in my education, even in the midst of this profound social values and social justice education, I can think back to spending my second year of field placement as a white student in a mostly African-American settlement house and never directly dealing with the inter-ethnic and social class issues between myself and my clients that were just below the surface. I know that my display of caring and concern for my clients allowed me to develop strong working relationships with many of the teenagers in the program. I know I was helpful, in my own sometimes bumbling way, as they indirectly addressed their issues of growing up in a racist society. However, I still regret the missed opportunities that resulted from my inability to understand, and my fear of making mistakes that kept me from confronting issues of race and class. As I will describe later, the struggle continues; however, I became better at catching my mistakes.

THE MIDDLE YEARS: EXPERIMENTING, LEARNING FROM MISTAKES AND MAKING MORE SOPHISTICATED MISTAKES

I have grown to understand that professional development is a life long process. I have tried to encourage my students, participants in my training workshops, and readers of my texts and articles not to be too harsh on themselves as they look back on mistakes they have made. I explain that they have probably been more helpful than they thought, even though in retrospect, they could think of more effective interventions. If they avoided a taboo issue related to the group or to a core concern of the members, and they recognized this and raised it at the next group meeting, they were skillful practitioners with a reasonably short distance between making a mistake and catching it. Even longer distances (a number of sessions later) were still OK. Even if the group was long gone, I encouraged them to "hang the painting" and admire what they had done well and reflect, with hind sight, on what they would do differently with the next opportunity on the next "canvass." I reassured them not to worry because additional opportunities would present themselves.

Even better, I encouraged them to take risks and to trust their feelings. I suggested that contrary to much of our professional training, we are better off introducing more spontaneity into our practice than waiting to be sure of saying the right thing. My research and experience taught me that we tend to make more mistakes of omission (failing to trust ourselves) than we do mistakes of commission (taking a risk and being wrong) (Shulman, 1988). If, for example, I was sensing the group was hinting at a difficult and taboo area of work, but I was unsure how to open the discussion or where it would go, I would want to trust this instinct and say: "A part of me feels you are really raising a very painful area about events in your life that can trigger your drinking, but another part of me is not sure how to make it safe for you to discuss it or in what direction the conversation will go."

By expressing this feeling of ambivalence, by putting it into words and identifying the taboo area, I would be modeling taking a risk as well as a caring sensitivity to the concerns of the clients. Once again, my research and experience have taught me in these middle years that this is how one develops the courage and skill. We need to learn how to use our feelings, not lose our feelings. As we open up taboo areas, often by expressing feelings that mirror those of our group members, or modeling for our group members a willingness to take a risk, our comfort in addressing these taboo areas grows. As we see our groups develop a culture that is more fearless, supportive and caring, our confidence continues to grow and we take more risks. We also observe the resilience of the group, its members and ourselves. Initial responses may include heightened defensiveness, denial, anger and increased avoidance; however, our willingness to persist, to send the message that we are ready when they are ready, will often lead to the breakthroughs that shatter the illusion of work and lead to profound growth for all concerned.

In the early years of my practice, I remember vividly a discussion group I led in a summer camp for disabled children and adults. It was a daily "current events discussion" group. One afternoon, the members chose to discuss a newspaper article that first exposed the connection between Thalidomide and birth defects. The group was diverse with members who were deformed at birth, others who struggled with the effects of muscular dystrophy or cerebral palsy and a group who had been disabled from Polio or an accident. All sat each day in their wheel chairs, arranged in a circle, to discuss the day's current events.

I could sense something was different almost from the start as the subgroup members who were disabled later in life, all agreed that it would have been better for these Thalidomide babies to die at birth than to live deformed. The response from one of the members with cerebral palsy, who was often almost violently spastic and spoke only with great difficulty, was angry and as immediately as his speech allowed, he asked if they thought he also should have died at birth, because although he didn't look like he had much going for him, he would have wanted to live. As a group leader, not expecting or prepared for this anger, I felt almost as paralyzed as my members. The tensions eased as other group members moved into the discussion to try to decrease the sense of confrontation. While one taboo, the rule against confrontation and expressions of anger had fallen, other taboos were still in place and I missed the opportunity to address them.

I have often replayed that group session. In fact the whole summer and my two years employed full-time at the sponsoring agency, I regretted I had not had the skill and courage to open up a discussion of what all of the group members felt about their physical disabilities and being short changed by life. It would have been helpful if I could have opened up the issues for paraplegics and quadriplegics who must have felt the sudden change in their life status. For many of the men, it was their pain at no longer feeling like "real men" and their loss of what they felt should have been their normal lives as partners, husbands and fathers. I later learned that their deeply felt feelings of shame and depreciated self-image often emerged as their desire to distinguish themselves from those who were born "cripples."

How helpful it would have been if I could have helped my extremely intelligent and well-educated cerebral palsied adult share his pain at being judged by his appearance. Family members and others who didn't take the time to listen because they assumed he had nothing to say or it was just too difficult to understand. It would have been important to help all the group members identify their common ground, address the institutional barriers and social stereotypes and oppression that added to their struggles to lead productive lives. Legislation would come later to address some of these social policy issues, but at this time most of us, including this social worker, did not really understand nor have the courage to explore these taboo issues. I could now deal with anger in the group, but I still struggled with the underlying pain.

THE LATER YEARS:
THE LEARNING CONTINUES

I vividly remember leading a Friday and Saturday workshop on group work at a University for about 150 participants. I was uncomfortable the first day, feeling the room was not very conducive to my training. We rearranged chairs to allow for more active participation, but I know I was a bit upset at the room selected by the Continuing Education staff. As the day progressed, we had difficulty with the heating and cooling system and were not able to get anyone from the custodial staff to properly set the thermostat.

The training itself was going well in spite of the physical conditions. It consisted of a combination of my presentations illustrated by examples, some of which I shared and others were detailed examples shared by participants. The first day dealt with issues of beginning and contracting, the individual in the group (e.g., deviant members, scapegoats) and a beginning discussion of how to help a group develop a culture for work. Some examples shared the first day and others placed on the agenda for the second day included dealing with "inter-ethnic" (between groups) and "intra-ethnic" (within groups) differences, and how they affected the group. We had one example of a white worker dealing with a group composed of members-of-color scheduled for discussion on the second day's agenda. It was offered by a worker in response to my encouraging this area of discussion and doing some preparatory work with the group on the tendency to avoid discussions in the area of race. The participants in the workshop were themselves diverse and seemed to respond positively, although somewhat nervously, to my suggestions about how we could address potentially toxic or difficult areas.

With so many participants it was hard to recognize everyone or even to have them all introduce themselves. On the second day, a Saturday session, we started at nine. Most of the participants were dressed in "weekend" clothes. The temperature in the room was very warm. I called to the custodial staff and they promised to have someone come and adjust the setting. About forty minutes into the session, an African-American male dressed in a sweatshirt and baseball cap appeared at the door and seemed to be looking around the crowded room. Relieved, I welcomed him and told him the thermostat was on the far wall. He thanked me for welcoming him and then told me he was not the custodian. He was a participant and was sorry he was late.

I still remember the sweat breaking out on my forehead. I remember vividly the sinking feeling I had as I realized I had assumed he was a maintenance man, and that it would be difficult for me to convince even myself that his race had nothing to do with it. With over thirty years of experience under my belt, having taught and written about how to deal with such situations, I immediately dropped the subject and returned to the example and the discussion we had been involved in. We continued to work, but I felt increasingly uncomfortable. Out of the corner of my eye, I had seen the four African-American women in the first row briefly glance at each other when I had made the mistake. The work proceeded, but I knew in my heart it was an illusion of work. The whole workshop group conspired to continue the workshop as if nothing happened.

At last, following my own advice (and feeling a bit desperate), just before the morning break, I said I wanted to discuss what had happened when Jim had entered and I had assumed he was the maintenance man. I could feel a collective sigh of relief as well as some holding of breaths. I described in detail my feelings at the earlier moment, how I had known it was important to acknowledge and discuss the incident, but that I had just tried to put my head down and plow ahead. I said that was a mistake and apologized, recognizing that this was part of the larger problem people of color faced as assumptions were made based upon appearances.

The response was electric as the whole group came alive with a discussion from the perspective of the participants of color as well as the white group members. The four African-American women in the first row laughed and told me they had wondered if I was going to address it or duck it. They were glad I had raised it. Examples of avoidance of the issue of racial issues, by both subgroups, the white workers and workers-of-color, as they attempted to lead their own client groups were shared. I asked participants to keep the conversation closely connected to the purpose of the workshop, focussing on leading mutual aid support groups. Powerful work continued on issues that had been taboo for most of the members. One of the participants commented that I had said at the start of the workshop on Friday that I would try to "practice what I preached" and that they had just seen an example of what I meant. I told them I had to be continually reminded that more was "caught" by participants than "taught" by the group leader, and that it would have been ironic to lead a workshop addressing taboo issues if I had modeled just the opposite. On reflection, I once again realized how false the dichotomy is between "process" and "content." By dealing with the example in that workshop, I had done some of my best teaching. I was "catching my mistake" and trusting my feelings during the session, which by my definition was the sign of a more sophisticated use of skill.

A RECENT PRACTICE EXAMPLE: CONFRONTING TABOOS WITH RECOVERING ADDICTS WITH AIDS

The example is drawn from the fifth session of a group I co-led for persons with AIDS in early substance abuse recovery. At the start of the session, I confronted the group members with their pattern of avoiding any discussion of AIDS and instead focusing on the more comfortable issues related to recovery. I pointed out that this appeared to be a taboo subject. Theresa responded by sharing an incident with her boy friend, whom she felt was flirting with another woman in front of her. While

Theresa presented a very real and painful problem, she had still not focused on her illness even though she said at the start of the session that she wanted to address it. I was conscious of this as I tried to explore with her and the group why she had accepted the current situation with her boyfriend. I was making what Schwartz (1961) had described as a "demand for work" and what I have called a facilitative confrontation (Shulman, 1999). It was a gentle demand in which I asked Theresa to examine her reasons for not pursuing the issues.

> I asked Theresa why she let her boy friend back off when she asked him to talk about his losses and her AIDS. She said, "Well, he told me it was hard to talk about." I responded, "Well, you could have asked him what made it hard. Why do you give up when he resists conversations with you?" There was a long silence and then Theresa's face softened and she said, "I guess I really don't want to hear." Everyone in the room nodded their head in agreement. I said, "Good for you, Theresa. Now you're taking some responsibility. What are you afraid you're going to hear?" She went on and said, "I'm afraid I'm going to be rejected."

> Jake jumped in at that point, with a lot of emotion, and described a court appearance at which his mother told the Judge he had AIDS. He went on to talk about how he didn't want people to know about his AIDS and that he felt rejection and shame from his own mother. The court sentenced him to jail, he believed, because of his AIDS.

> Tania had been very quiet, although I could tell she wanted to speak. At one point, I said, "I think Tania wants to get in here, and she's been well-behaved this session, we have to give her a chance." She smiled and jumped in, telling Theresa how much she admired her, and how much strength she had, and that she hoped that she could handle her own recovery in the way that Theresa was handling hers. She told Theresa that she just deserved a lot more.

> Theresa asked Tania whether she thought she was an attractive person. There was a silence and Tania said, "I think you're a beautiful young woman and you could have any man you want." Theresa went on at some length about how men come on to her and, if she wanted to, she could "bump and grind" with them as well. But she didn't want that. She wanted one relationship. She

wanted a serious relationship. She said she was getting older now and she wanted a commitment from someone and this was just not enough, and that was what the issue was all about.

Jake, our often quiet yet very thoughtful member had changed the norm and broken the taboo by raising the fear of rejection associated with AIDS. Theresa's question to Tania about her looks was an indirect way of getting at the issue of fear of rejection. I tried in the next excerpt to facilitate her expression by articulating her feelings.

I said to Theresa, "Is the question really that you're afraid that he might not stay with you, that if you actually confront him on this issue of the other women, that he might leave you?" She agreed that it was her concern. At this point, I wondered if it might help Theresa to figure out what she might say to her boyfriend. Theresa said that would be helpful because she didn't know when and how to say it. Then she laughed and said, "Maybe I should say it in bed." Tania said, "Oh no. Don't say it before sex and don't say it after sex." And I added, "And don't say it during sex." Everyone laughed and Tania did a hilarious imitation of having a conversation with Theresa's boyfriend, while pumping up and down as if she were in bed having sex with him.

After the laughter died down, Tania said, "You have to find a quiet time, not a time when you're in the middle of a fight, and you have to just put out your feelings." I asked Tania if she could show Theresa how she could do that. She started to speak as if she were talking to Theresa's boyfriend. I role-played the boyfriend.

Theresa listened carefully and then said, "I know I have to talk to him, but, you know, he told me that he's not sure he wants to be tied down, that he likes to have his freedom." Jake nodded his head and said, "Yeah, that's the problem, they want their freedom and they don't want to make a commitment, and you're afraid, if you push him, he'll leave you because you've got the virus." Theresa said she realized she had to sit down and talk to him because it couldn't keep up the same way. She would just get too angry and do something crazy and screw up her recovery. She felt she had to find another way to get through to him and talk to him. Otherwise, this thing was just going to continue and it was going to tear her up inside.

I said, if she did confront him, it was going to be very rough for her, especially with the holiday, and I wondered whom she'd have for support, especially if he said he didn't want to continue the relationship. She said she had her sponsor, and Tania said, "You also have me. You can call me anytime you want." Tania said, "I didn't realize when I started this group there were people who have lived lives just like me, who had feelings just like me, who had struggles just like me. You–you're a woman–you've really helped me see that I'm just not the only one going through this. I'd do anything I could to help you."

Once again, Theresa asked Tania how she looked. She said, "You're a woman. I know, as a woman, you will be honest with me and just tell me what you think. Do you think I look okay?" Tania seemed confused and said, "Well, sure, you look wonderful." I said, "I wonder if Theresa is really asking, "Am I pretty enough? Am I attractive enough? If my boyfriend leaves me, can I find someone else who could love me even though I have AIDS?," She said, "That's it," and started to cry. She said, "I'm so afraid, if I lose him, I won't find anyone else." She said, "I know I could have guys, and I know I could have sex, and I like the sex. I sure missed it during the time I was in prison, but can another guy love me?"

CONCLUSION

I hope my brief description of my professional journey is helpful to the reader. I have learned that to be effective as a group worker I must continue to grow. Whoever said that there was growth from pain knew what they were talking about. I think my practice and teaching (and my current work as a Dean) has been aided by my willingness to confront taboo subjects. I remember the words of one of my first year social work students who said, "But it sounds so easy when you say it." I know it is not easy and I wish there were some way to speed up the learning process. Unfortunately, there is no easy way. Each learner must make mistakes, learn from their mistakes, and make more sophisticated mistakes as they tackle the taboo issues that make up so much of our work.

BIBLIOGRAPHY

Schwartz, W. (1961). The social worker in the group. In *New perspectives on services to groups: Theory, organization, practice* (pp. 7-34). New York: National Association of Social Workers.

Schwartz, W. (1969). Private troubles and public issues: One social work job or two? In *The social welfare forum* (pp. 24-43). New York: Columbia University Press.

Shulman, L. (1988). Developing and testing a practice theory: The interactional perspective. *Social Work, 38*, 91-97.

Shulman, L. (1999). *The skills of helping individuals, families, communities and groups* (4th ed.). Itasca, IL: F. E. Peacock, Publishers.

My Love Affair
with Stages
of Group Development

Toby Berman-Rossi

The first social work group I remember working with was a girls' group in a community center. It was a fun socialization group. I loved working with the girls. We did all sorts of great things together. Though a long time ago, certain memories persist. These memories can be labeled my pre: knowledge of stages of group development days. I had no real understanding of group development and it never occurred to me there was any patterned rhythm to the development of my group. Both the girls and I were full of energy, though they of course had more. It seemed they could run through the halls forever and I would always have trouble keeping up. I had trouble keeping up in many ways. For example, the girls seemed to oppose and cooperate with me, at will. Just when I thought things were going well, an unexpected whammy would occur. No doubt their cooperative behavior was more pleasing to me and I did not understand their opposition. Sometimes their combativeness felt personal. That was hard to understand. How could they view me as an oppressive authority? I was only 17 at the time. Their behavior seemed very much on their terms and the group seemed to have a life of its own. When things didn't work or the process didn't go well, as a beginning worker I personalized everything. After all, I was not very skilled or knowledgeable. Personalizing was often painful. Little did I

[Haworth co-indexing entry note]: "My Love Affair with Stages of Group Development." Berman-Rossi, Toby. Co-published simultaneously in *Social Work with Groups* (The Haworth Social Work Practice Press, an imprint of The Haworth Press, Inc.) Vol. 25, No. 1/2, 2002, pp. 151-158; and: *Stories Celebrating Group Work: It's Not Always Easy to Sit on Your Mouth* (ed: Roselle Kurland, and Andrew Malekoff) The Haworth Social Work Practice Press, an imprint of The Haworth Press, Inc., 2002, pp. 151-158. Single or multiple copies of this article are available for a fee from The Haworth Document Delivery Service [1-800-HAWORTH, 9:00 a.m. - 5:00 p.m. (EST). E-mail address: getinfo@haworthpressinc.com].

know at the time that "the authority theme" would become a major focus in my practice.

In social work camp, over the next three summers, I had some intense experiences with groups. Every three weeks children would leave and arrive. These, too, were part of my "pre-days." I could tell the groups were not all the same but I had no tools for understanding their character or for thinking about my group work with the children. We had lots of training and good social work group supervision, and there was a good deal of mutual aid among the counselors, but I still lacked a framework for understanding my bunks (cabin groups) as a whole. Clearly, some groups seemed to jell and others seemed never to get there. Some groups challenged my authority, directly and hard, while others appeared more cooperative, and the members appeared more concerned with where they stood with each other. Occasionally the same groups did both. That was especially confusing.

What also struck me was that sometimes my groups behaved differently under different circumstances. For example, when the camp had its final Festival of Nations and each bunk had to present the music, dance, song, and customs of a different country, sometimes the group members pulled together and transcended their differences and sometimes a bunk stayed stuck, mired in its difficulties, arguing over everything. I wondered what would prompt one group to band together in mutual aid and another to be unable to move forward, despite all my best efforts. Another puzzling thing I noticed was that while there was often consistency between how the children behaved with me individually and how they behaved in the bunk, there often were differences. The child I thought I had a good relationship with individually would sometimes oppose me publicly when we were together with the others, and the children I didn't think I had such a close relationship with individually would often support me. Most confusing!

Often I felt bumped about by my groups. I certainly did not understand the members' opposition or their "ganging" up on me. When I did try to understand, my frame of reference was family. I reasoned that maybe I was like a parent to them. In a sense this was true, of course. I was the one to tell them what they could and couldn't do. I was the one who tucked them in at night, read them stories, and offered good night kisses. What was not true was that their behavior was all about me. My reactions were too personal and too individualized to be entirely helpful. While what I did surely mattered, it was not the whole story.

"The whole story" was something I learned about in social work school. In those days (1963-1965), practice methods were separated and one had to choose. Happily, I chose both casework and group work. My group work classes and group work teachers (William Schwartz and Irving Miller) were especially instructive. The knowledge I gained was transformative, personally and professionally. Many ideas stand out, but professional function, group purpose, skill, mutual aid, and stages of group development have had enduring value for me as a practitioner, field instructor, supervisor, and educator. Taken together, these five ideas combined to provide a powerful foundation and direction for my practice with groups.

Eight methods courses (four in casework and four in group work) allowed for a more leisurely examination of core ideas. Even then we believed each course covered too much. In Groups II we were introduced to the far reaching concept of the group as a whole. Though the notion that the group as a whole is greater than the sum of its parts was an idea we experienced in our everyday lives, it was a new and powerful idea to us as social work students. We studied not only psychological theories of how groups developed (e.g., Bennis and Shepard, 1956; Bion, 1961; Freud, 1922/1959) (Garland, Jones, and Kolodny had not yet published their germinal work), but sociological theories as well (e.g., Homans, 1950; Olmstead, 1959).

We learned much. First there was the shared belief that groups develop over time and that there were differing explanations for that development (psychological and sociological). We learned that group development was not random, but rather it was patterned and that different theorists saw different patterns, e.g., linear-progressive, life-cycle, pendular, and offered different explanations for these patterns. From psychological theories we learned about "the authority theme" and "the intimacy theme" (Bennis and Shepard). Sociological theories offered us concepts such as norms, culture, cliques, social ranking, and the interdependence of interaction and sentiment, patterns of association (Homans; Olmstead). All ideas expanded our knowledge base. At first we didn't understand how knowledge of stages of group development would expand our practice base as well, but we would learn.

Several aspects of psychological theories caught my attention. Bennis and Shepard's (1956) idea that the "resolution" of the authority relationship between the worker and the members preceded the development of intimacy among members was an enormously powerful idea for me. Ah . . . there was a predictability to the power struggle in my groups. For the first time I had a theoretical basis for believing that such struggles were not all my fault. Unfortunately, my relief was only temporarily comforting. Was it true that no matter what I did, such struggles would ensue? The prospect of endless power struggles was not encouraging. Nor was it heartening to believe that skill mattered so little. After all, why labor so hard in the Record of Service, or the Critical Incident Analysis, if my professional action could not alter the development of my groups? And how could I grab a hold of the idea that more developed groups were more satisfying to members and more readily helped them do the work for which they were gathered, if I couldn't alter my group's development?

My struggles filled pages in my Groups II log. It was out of these struggles that some of my most important learning about group development occurred. I badgered my teacher. Luckily, my pushing and questioning and challenging did not phase Professor Schwartz. He had been down this road before and knew it was coming. He knew that I (and others) had been harboring an all or nothing conception of group development. It felt to us that we either controlled all of our groups' development or we influenced none of it. He knew that we had yet to fully appreciate the nature of the group as a whole. He knew I had to replace the concept of control with the concept of influence. I didn't sufficiently understand that the group as a whole had its own identity, energy, and power for growth and development and that only by joining with that energy could our power relationships be sufficiently resolved for the group to move on in its development. Although I could articulate the idea of partnership, I didn't really understand that I believed in a notion of partnership on my terms. Moving toward true partnership was initially frightening but ultimately liberating for both the group and myself. It was within this idea of an alliance between the group and myself that I began to get a glimmer of my function as a social worker.

It was toward the end of Groups II that theories of group development, professional function, group purpose, skill, and mutual aid began to come together a little. (Happily, I had another year of group work for it to come together more.) My theoretical guardedness shifted to studying the nature of my influence within the group. I moved from "whether" to "how" and in so moving the convergence of these five critical factors finally took on the interdependent meaning they deserved. The questions now became how do I help my groups develop; what skills do I use; what's the division of labor between the members and myself in achieving group development. This last question brought me full circle to the concept of professional function and group purpose. I had work to do and the members had work to do. It was my job was to help them do their work and realize the purpose for which they had come together. The more skillful I was, the more helpful I would be in helping the members work. As well, if I could help the group as a whole develop, it too would strengthen the members' abilities to get the work done.

I felt ready for practice upon graduation. Of course I had much more to learn but I had a sense of preparedness. My first job on the adolescent unit of a large, milieu therapy based, psychiatric hospital would test that sense of preparedness. It was here that I was afforded the opportunity to use my knowledge and skills to further formulate my thinking about practice. As a group worker, I worked with groups morning, afternoon, and evening. There were new patient orientation groups, roommate groups, program planning groups, evening activity groups, new family orientation groups, ongoing family groups, weekend pass groups, government groups, executive committee groups, community trip groups, pre-discharge groups and various spontaneous groups. I was awash in patient and staff groups. Though I sometimes groaned under the weight of almost as many staff and team meetings as patient meetings, it was that total immersion in collective endeavors that fostered the development of my thinking.

I saw that stages of group development theory applied everywhere. New insights were generated for my systems work as well as for my practice with the girls and their families. Actual experience affirmed that no matter how good the theory, its use and application were up to me. Many of the psychological theories concerned time-limited, close-ended groups. My groups were long-term and open-ended. While they didn't quite fit the model, they were close enough. On the whole, changes in membership were few and only occurred monthly. By and large my groups fit Galinsky and Schopler's (1985, 1989) Type 4 groups, the type of open-ended group most capable of group development.

The girls seemed to take new admissions in stride. With only one or two admissions a month, there was time and emotional energy available to integrate new members. My arrival was more unsettling for the girls and had a significant impact on the groups as a whole. At our first group meeting they boasted of having chased away my predecessor. The hurt in the bravado was palpable. Their continuous and unrelenting testing was difficult to take. It felt as if nothing I did was good enough. Staff's behavior toward me mirrored the girls' behavior. Thankfully, the staff's testing period was shorter and not quite as virulent. Over time (the girls stayed an average of 18 months and I stayed nearly five years), the challenging gave way to signs that the group as a whole had moved toward greater intimacy. Preoccupation with my authority lessened and the work among the girls became more intimate. Differences were more readily accepted. The groups as a whole provided sustaining support and I learned that the stronger they were, the more they offered the group members.

I was still learning the skills of strengthening the group as a whole when I changed jobs. For the next 15 years I worked in a long-term care facility for older persons. Here too I worked with myriad resident, family, and staff groups. My previous work had primed me to expect lots of challenging and testing behavior. To my surprise the opposite occurred as I assumed the role of group worker on five floors. Group members were quite deferential. The flip side of "the authority theme" now appeared. Here it seemed, by and large, I could do no wrong. Of course this was not true for every person, every time, but most saw me as a sweet granddaughter whom they did not want to challenge. My practice shifted from engaging attacks to helping the members take on my authority and power. Over time I came to better recognize the subtlety of the challenges and over time the residents became more comfortable being direct.

My new experiences prompted me to further develop my thinking about group development. It was now patently obvious that all of my groups did not develop in the same manner. Clearly there were major differences in the development of my adolescent groups and my groups of older persons. And . . . even within each setting there were developmental differences. No doubt there was more "feistiness" in my new patient admission group and more intimacy in my pre-discharge adolescent group. The leadership training group in the long-term care facility firmly held its ground, while much deferring occurred in the new residents group. Perhaps stages of group development were not universally the same for all groups. How then to make sense of the dominant paradigm that was so clearly articulated by Garland, Jones, and Kolodny (1965)? Like others, I was appreciative of the ideas and created variations on the theory to fit my particular groups.

Moving into teaching provided a new vantage point for understanding group development and for the further development of my skill. Every class was a group and each session would reflect my practice with a group. Of course, class groups and client groups were not identical but each had work to do and each had a social worker whose function it was to help the members do the work for which they were gathered. How exciting and challenging to experience the parallel process at work. As we learned from shared experiences, the learning became richly enhanced. Each classroom group then became a partnership in the teaching-learning experience.

It is now 43 years since my first musings about group development. Without question, the subject has held my attention. I remain convinced that the stronger the group as a whole, the better able are members to realize the purpose for which they have gathered. I remain resolute in my belief that the small group really is the building block of democratic society and that our work in strengthening the group as a whole fundamentally strengthens individuals, communities, and society at large.

It remains exciting that as much as we know, there is more to study and more to know. No doubt, gender (Schiller, 1995, 1997), structure, patterns of attendance, content, context and population (age, vulnerability, dependence), and worker skill (Kelly and Berman-Rossi, 1999), diversity and the societal context (Garvin and Reed, 1994) and much more, have bearing on the development of our groups. I feel moved that we remain committed to studying the factors that bear on group development and to the skills of strengthening the resiliency of the group as a whole. To continue this dedication is to sustain the mission of our profession.

REFERENCES

Bennis, W. and Shepard, H. (1956). A theory of group development. *Human relations.* 9, 415-457.

Bion, W. R. (1961). *Experiences in groups.* New York: Ballantine Books.

Freud, S. (1959). *Group psychology and the analysis of the ego.* Translated and edited by J. Strachey. New York: W. W. Norton & Co. Original published in 1922.

Galinsky, M. J., and Schopler, J. H. (1989). Developmental patterns in open-ended groups. *Social Work with Groups,* 12 (2), 99-114.

Galinsky, M. and Schopler, J. (1985). Patterns of entry and exit in open-ended groups. *Social Work with Groups,* 8 (2), 67-80.

Garland, J., Jones, H. and Kolodny, R. (1965). A model of stages of development in social group work groups. In S. Bernstein, (Ed.), *Explorations in group work.* (pp. 12-53). Boston: Boston University School of Social Work.

Garvin, C. and Reed, B. (1994). Small group theory and social work practice: Promoting diversity and social justice or recreating inequities? In R. R. Greene (Ed.), *Human behavior theory: A diversity framework.* (pp. 173-202). New York: Aldine de Gruyter.

Homan, G. C. (1950). *The human group.* New York: Harcourt, Brace and World.

Kelly, T. B. and Berman-Rossi, T. (1999). Advancing stages of group development theory: The case of institutionalized older persons. *Social Work with Groups,* 22 (2/3), 119-138.

Olmstead, M. S. (1959). *The small group*. New York: Random House.

Schiller, L. (1995). Stages of development in women's groups: A relational model. In R. Kurland and R. Salmon (Eds.), *Group work practice in a troubled society: Problems and opportunities*, pp. 117-138. New York: The Haworth Press, Inc.

Schiller, L. (1997). Rethinking stages of development in women's groups: Implications for practice. *Social Work with Groups,* 20 (3), 3-19.

Process of an Idea–
How the Relational Model
of Group Work Developed

Linda Yael Schiller

What if what I had learned about groups in social work school was wrong–at least some of the time? And who was I anyway to challenge the prevailing wisdom?

I had this fairly radical thought early one very cold winter morning in November 1993. I was driving on route 128 on my way to present a workshop about survivors of sexual abuse to an agency on the North Shore, and I had just joined the faculty at Boston University as a part-time professor a year or two ago. I remember that I had the heater on high, and the windows were just finishing defrosting; little rivulets of water were inching their way down the glass. As I negotiated the rush hour traffic I was thinking about the groups I had been running for the past several years, in particular the current one that I had been running with a co-leader for abuse survivors.

Most of my groups didn't usually seem to follow the format I had learned in social work school regarding the stages of group develop-ment. In fact, the women in many of my groups didn't really get into any conflict at all until much later on in the group, and never really went through the "power and control" stage I had learned about. My current group of female abuse survivors was in its tenth meeting out of a total of sixteen. The members had been consistently supportive of each other and hadn't given the workers a hard time at all; contrary to what the

[Haworth co-indexing entry note]: "Process of an Idea–How the Relational Model of Group Work Developed." Schiller, Linda Yael. Co-published simultaneously in *Social Work with Groups* (The Haworth Social Work Practice Press, an imprint of The Haworth Press, Inc.) Vol. 25, No. 1/2, 2002, pp. 159-166; and: *Stories Celebrating Group Work: It's Not Always Easy to Sit on Your Mouth* (ed: Roselle Kurland, and Andrew Malekoff) The Haworth Social Work Practice Press, an imprint of The Haworth Press, Inc., 2002, pp. 159-166. Single or multiple copies of this article are available for a fee from The Haworth Document Delivery Service [1-800-HAWORTH, 9:00 a.m. - 5:00 p.m. (EST). E-mail address: getinfo@haworthpressinc.com].

159

"power and control" stage part of group development theory would have us believe. The biggest conflict we had with the group thus far was around who would go first when the story sharing part of the group was coming up; which was less about any conflict and more a function of member anxiety and their desire to not be too assertive about their owns needs or desires ("No, you go first, it's really O.K., I can wait till another week").

However, in spite of this deviation from standard social work group practice, the group seemed to be going well and members reported satisfaction and growth. My co-leader and I had been talking about this phenomenon, and I had mentioned it to several other colleagues at the agency I was currently working at, a community trauma and sexual abuse center. They said that they had frequently observed the same thing, but didn't have any explanation for it either, and were frankly relieved not to have to deal with much conflict in their groups. Some were counting it as a bonus if their groups stayed "nice" throughout, especially those who were also running kids' groups, where conflict management was the order of the day. The other groups I had been facilitating had a variety of purposes and formats over the years, but the common variable in most of them was that the members were all women.

As I pulled off the highway, I suddenly had a flash: What if there is a different model for women's groups? I had recently read some of Carol Gilligan's work, and the first book of a compilation of working papers from the Stone Center at Wellesley College about the new relational model of psychological development for women. There was an abundance of new scholarship about women's psychological growth and development, much of it stressing women's ability and need for connection as a hallmark of growth, but none of it had touched on this developmental variation for groups, as far as I could tell. Ideas about women's seeming avoidance of conflict and need for connections began to flood into my head. It actually was one of those "ah-ha" moments, when several things seemed to come together, like the click when you hit the last number on the combination lock.

I began to think about other groups that I had facilitated or was a member of. As I pulled up to the agency, I parked the car and scrambled in my briefcase for a piece of paper that didn't already contain lecture notes or other items of importance. I came up with the back of my grocery list, and jotted down in short order "establishing a relational base" and "challenge and change," and then got stuck as to what to call the additional stage that seemed to come between these two. I needed to go in to give the workshop at this point, which included some ideas for working with survivors in groups. On the way home, I played with some headings for this elusive middle stage. They got scribbled on the same grocery list, but I was driving this time, and had to then decipher my handwriting when I got home. I finally settled on "Mutuality and interpersonal empathy" as the best descriptive title I could come up with. (It has always felt a bit unwieldy to me however; not as succinct or catchy as the other two.) So now the names of the five stages that I felt were descriptive of women's group development were (1) Pre-affiliation, (2) Establishing a Relational Base, (3) Mutuality and Interpersonal Empathy, (4) Challenge and Change, and (5) Separation and Termination.

My next step was to write up a brief outline of my thoughts and ideas about this new concept, and take them in to show Larry Shulman, who was my sequence chair of the group work department at Boston University School of Social Work at the time. I remember feeling some trepidation, for as the new kid on the block, I didn't want to step on any toes. In particular, I was aware that Boston University was "group development central," and that the prevailing model of stages of group development was inseminated here. In addition, at this stage of my participation in the group known as the group work faculty staff meetings, I could rarely get a word in edgewise. I remember this as feeling out of the norm of my usual style in groups, which is usually to be quite active and verbal. My relative silence was mostly because of my awe at sitting at the same table as the "big boys," my previous teachers, and also because the male personalities in the room tended to quickly fill up the allotted time.

Once Larry was intrigued with my ideas, he suggested that I show my work to Jim Garland. I was concerned about showing it to Jim, however, because I didn't want him to feel insulted that I had proposed a variation on his (along with Ralph Kolodny and Hubie Jones) model. To my relief, Jim was supportive from the start; he returned the paper to me marked up with enthusiastic comments. Either Jim or Larry, or maybe both, encouraged me to submit a proposal to the AASWG conference coming up in New York the next fall.

Over the next few months I fleshed out the ideas and added examples to illustrate the points. In the summer, the Massachusetts AASWG board invited me down to their annual summer retreat to talk about my relational model of stages of group development. There I got an opportunity to present the model publicly for the first time. I could feel the members' interest and their hesitancy as I spoke, and the first responses were tentative and somewhat challenging. After all, Jim was sitting right there and people weren't sure what he was making of all this. Also, this was a group of men, and I've learned over the years of public speaking that women often show their interest or support with head nodding and smiles, while men frequently show their interest by asking challenging questions. But Jim chimed in with his endorsement and support, and said that he felt that this was a way of actually keeping the original model alive.

I didn't have an actual paper when I went to the New York City AASWG conference, just lecture notes. I had a fair amount of experience teaching by now and usually wasn't nervous, but this time I was. I felt that not only would I not be teaching to students, or even just to my peers, but also potentially to my teachers, the ones who wrote the books and articles I had learned from. I even asked Jim not to come to my workshop, but he assured me that he would be on his best behavior and not put me on the spot. He actually sat on the floor in the back of the room since it was quite crowded, so I couldn't see him at all as I spoke, much to my relief. A week or so later I received a call from Roselle Kurland, telling me that they would like to have my paper included in the edited collection of selected papers from that conference. I don't think I realized until this point that these ideas might be something relevant to a much broader audience. Since I only had lecture notes up until now, the invitation to be included in the publication meant that I had to turn it into an actual article, complete with footnotes and correct spelling. (Thank God for spell check!)

One example of where some of these ideas came from, particularly around women and conflict, comes from a group of which I have been a member for about ten years, my dream circle. This is a leaderless group of four or five women that comes together monthly for potluck dinner and to work on our dreams with each other. As I recall, it took about three years before any overt conflict surfaced between us (that's right, years!). I'm pretty sure that the leaderless format of our group is what kept us circling an issue as long as we did; we needed some good strong facilitation to be more comfortable with dealing directly with conflict.

And the member who was having the difficulty with another member told us that she had been talking to her therapist about how to bring it up to the group for several months before she finally did so. We all struggled with the tension the issue raised, and I remember feeling uncomfortable, even though the conflict did not involve me directly. She ultimately made the decision to leave the group because she "didn't want to cause any more tension for the group"; in spite of the fact that she was the one who had brought the idea of the dream circle to us and had put the group together. I remember feeling sad that we hadn't been able to find a way to enable her to stay and still feel safe. We added another member, and in this new configuration it was another five or six years before the next tense issue came up.

This long time span between conflicts was in part due to who we all were individually and the type of connection we had to each other before joining the dream group, but there were also times when one or another of us clearly shied away from a hot button topic in the service of preserving the peace, myself included. The next time conflict surfaced, I was part of the equation. I clearly remember a choice point where I had said something that I know another member had misinterpreted and reacted to non-verbally, but hadn't brought up. I could easily have ignored it, but made an internal decision not to let it go. I remember mustering up my own courage to say, "It seems like you had a reaction to what I just said." It definitely took all of my courage at that moment to raise it; some years ago I probably would have just let it go. Her response was to breathe an audible sigh of relief and say, "I'm so glad you noticed, because I wouldn't have said anything." We continued with a painful but important discussion that I think ultimately brought us closer, and no one left the group this time.

By the time the first article was published in 1995, I had time to think about the theoretical concepts further, and realized that there were some practice implications for us as facilitators of these groups if they were developing along a different pathway. This time I did go straight to the article format, having gotten my feet wet with the first two (the stages model and a previous one I had co-authored on groups for sexual abuse survivors). The second article came out in 1997, with the emphasis on what facilitators of women's groups may want to rethink about their intervention styles as they work with these groups based on my experiences both as a facilitator and as a member of groups.

A few key points in that article included (1) Spending more time on explicitly establishing both safety and commonality among members, (2) A less hierarchical approach to facilitating that includes more of a flow of mutuality of affect between both members and facilitators and more worker self disclosure of response to the material being raised by members, and (3) Especially rethinking a traditionally less active role during the fourth stage for a much more active re-engagement in facilitation during the challenging time that members actively deal with conflict.

I began to present these ideas in various forums, and then was asked by the Florida AASWG chapter to also present any new ideas that I had at that time about applications of the model. Since I was now a new parent (having recently brought our daughter Sara home from China), I hadn't really done much more thinking about it. My intellectual creativity had been more taken up with finding good childcare, researching all-terrain strollers, and dusting off the verses to "Twinkle Twinkle Little Star" and "Old McDonald." So the invitation to present my "new ideas" generated an "uh-oh" feeling on my part. I wasn't sure that I had any new ideas since last time.

But as I thought about it, the feedback I had been receiving from students and colleagues indicated to me that this format of group development was likely applicable not only for women's groups, but also for many different types of groups that had members from vulnerable populations. Affiliation and connection preceding attention to difference, and connection through difference preceding connection in the face of conflict seemed to hold true for groups of many types where members were dealing with shame, displacement, trauma, disabilities, or oppression of various forms. These were part of what I presented at the Florida conference and continue to see as viable when I work and teach now. A sense of vulnerability, or of being "one-down," or feeling unsafe in the world or in one's neighborhood among group members can lead to group development along a relational line. Additionally, some cultures do not as brazenly stress independence as our American cowboy ethos does, and groups composed of Asian members, Native Americans, or other traditional cultures may prefer to proceed carefully and cautiously before engaging in conflict or disagreement, particularly when there are authority figures involved.

The flip side of a model of stages of development for women's groups is when the women's groups themselves don't seem to follow those stages. Some of my African American women students have told me that they think their peers would be much more apt to be "out there," and not hold back on challenging each other or authority right from the start. More often than not I find and hear of women's groups developing along the relational model, but clearly gender is only one of a host of variables that can influence the way a group develops. Race, ethnicity, age, social class, sexual orientation, presenting concern or problem, and worker experience are some of the others.

In fact, not only does worker experience, both with that particular population and with group work in general, make a difference regarding what happens in the group, I have begun to believe that it is one of the key variables that can actually influence how a group will develop. The worker's own personal orientation and philosophy, as well as intervention style and choices, can create an atmosphere that fosters group development along the lines of the relational model or along the lines of the traditional Boston model.

These ideas about the influence of the facilitator her/himself on how the group develops are expanded upon in a chapter in Marcia Cohen's and Audrey Mullender's book, *Gender and Groupwork,* which was due out in spring 2002. I have begun to see a difference between describing different models of group development in a descriptive fashion, or applying them in a proscriptive fashion. The later proscriptive use of stage theory is where the facilitator has made a conscious and clinical decision about which style or model would best serve the needs of the members of this particular group, given all its multiple variables, and then consciously working from that model.

Right now it is most definitely summer–(in contrast to beginning with defrosting windows) and I am waiting for my air conditioner to kick in. We're in what are affectionately known as the "dog days" of summer–it's 97 in the shade. My daughter is four now, and fell asleep in a heap for a rare nap after a long hot day at camp, enabling me to work on this article. At four, she doesn't have any problem speaking her mind or engaging in conflict whenever the mood strikes. She and her peers have usually forgotten all about it within five minutes, half an hour at the most. Watching them in the playground at her preschool sometimes reminds me of *Lord of the Flies,* but also of the solid roots for the Boston Model of group development. Power and Control is the name of the game here, ephemerally flowing in and out of true intimacy and connection as the children learn to negotiate their world.

Both the traditional Boston Model and the Relational Model have their strengths. Somewhere along the road of maturation, a shift happens. How we relate to each other as group members changes–because of nature, nurture, or a combination of the two. Acquiring more civility, subtlety and empathy allows for a greater safety and a deeper relational connection prior to engaging in conflict. The traditional model more quickly delves into conflict, perhaps clearing the air and forging the connections out of the resolution of the conflict. The goal of both is to establish connections among members and a system of mutual aid in the group that allow the work of the group to be accomplished.

As facilitators, our task remains to help all our group members to relate to and from their authentic selves regardless of gender, age, race, or vulnerabilities. Having self awareness of our own biases and orientation, as well as the flexibility to embrace the developmental model that seems right for this particular combination of members and then intervening accordingly, I believe, will help us to achieve dynamic and powerful groups for both members and workers alike.

For me, the ideas about group development came both from my professional life and from my personal life. I know that there are times when I step outside of myself in groups to watch what is going on–both as a facilitator and sometimes as a member, too (an occupational hazard, I guess). Having a very spirited preschool child forces me directly into the arena of conflict much more often than I would really care to be, but the good news is that it seems that I am at least having a "growth experience" because of it.

Group Work Is All Wet*
*Don't Read Article Until an Hour After Eating

Michael W. Wagner

What is it like to run a group? How do you do it? How do you keep control and get anything done? What do I need to know? What do I need to do? These are just the first questions, the tip of the iceberg for the student or the new group leader. Perhaps a field instructor or a supervisor has decided it would be good for them to do a group. Maybe their agency does all of its services in groups. In any case, the questions are full of anxious energy, hope and fear, but above all they are seeking a concise understanding of exactly what to do.

When most social work education takes the generalist practice form, the idea of doing social group work can become an almost foreign language for the learner. The casework interview, with its individual client, feels direct, almost surgical, in its application. My client says something, I say something, my client reacts and says another thing and I assess my intervention. If I can interpret effectively, I can help my client find solutions to problems of every day living. But in social group work every intervention is made to the collected group as much as it is to any individual client. My interpretations may be pre-empted by some response of another member. There is no surgical precision. It can feel as if my helping hands are cased in mittens, blunting my precision and foiling my interventions. The direct metaphors for helping seem inadequate to the task of describing social group work.

[Haworth co-indexing entry note]: "Group Work Is All Wet* *Don't Read Article Until an Hour After Eating." Wagner, Michael W. Co-published simultaneously in *Social Work with Groups* (The Haworth Social Work Practice Press, an imprint of The Haworth Press, Inc.) Vol. 25, No. 1/2, 2002, pp. 167-173; and: *Stories Celebrating Group Work: It's Not Always Easy to Sit on Your Mouth* (ed: Roselle Kurland, and Andrew Malekoff) The Haworth Social Work Practice Press, an imprint of The Haworth Press, Inc., 2002, pp. 167-173. Single or multiple copies of this article are available for a fee from The Haworth Document Delivery Service [1-800-HAWORTH, 9:00 a.m. - 5:00 p.m. (EST). E-mail address: getinfo@haworthpressinc.com].

167

Perhaps the frustration described above at working in the group sounds a bit familiar. I speak from my own experience with my first attempt at group services. In my first child welfare job I worked in a residential treatment facility for emotionally disturbed boys and girls, 4 to 11 years old. Residential treatment allowed for a great number of experiences working with the children in groups, but it is interesting that I recall doing very little social group work. I remember developing individual relationships as my main strategy to help them in the milieu of the treatment program. At my agency we opened a specialized day treatment program for our most disruptive children. Using a highly structured activity program to promote external structure that could be, hopefully, internalized, the program had as a cornerstone component a daily group.

The group's purpose was to help members identify the behaviors that resulted in their assignment to the program, to talk about whether that behavior had worked for them, to brainstorm new alternative behaviors and to make a plan to use the new behavior in the future. Children had to attend at least two of these groups to be able to return to the regular living unit programs.

We had such great hopes for the group's success: that members would help one another sort through the difficulties of living at the center, that each would gain from the other's experiences, that they would grow and develop more connected and intimate relationships that would one day allow them to return to families and lives filled with promise. What it became, however, was a great example of casework in a group. One child at a time spoke, answering four questions from the staff members with short, canned answers so that they could "do their time" and get back to "normal" life. We had no idea how to help this ragtag bunch become a group. At times we weren't sure it would even be a good idea!

We began with the expectation that all of the members would sit together and process each person's issues at a time. It didn't take long to discover that the group wouldn't work that way and, not knowing any better, we quickly broke the group into a collection of individuals, went to each in turn and processed all of the members separately to contain the group, maintain control and achieve our purpose. It may have been a collection, but it certainly wasn't group. And as a result we never achieved the full potential of the program to promote development. The intervention felt so imprecise and seemed to create chaos in the members. We saw it as a failure. We had attempted to use that surgical helping metaphor with no success.

I would suggest that my experience teaches me that working with groups is like being in water. Like my first experience, getting in the turbulent water can sometimes feel like one is drowning, being dragged under the surface by the demands of the many members, struggling for direction and a way to the surface, getting frantic before realizing that to find the way up one must get the water quiet enough around us for a bubble trail to the surface. Interventions in the group aren't precise and surgical because they act on the group like our hands or tools on water. A motion on one side of the pool creates ripples of agreement or disagreement on the other. The facilitator scans to see the ripples interact with the members and then accentuates or blunts the waves that the members' motions then send back to the group. The waves amplify and dampen one another in a constantly moving and ever changing dance.

We "dive right in" to see how the group is working and we understand that the water must be disturbed, roughed up and choppy, for any movement to be accomplished. Change comes with the movement of the tides of time and growth, with waves that push members out of comfortable positions into new roles and that guide the whole group along the lines of its evolving purpose. Describing the skills of social group work in the language of this water metaphor provides a window for engaging others in the more contextual experiences we have in group.

Acting as a field instructor or a supervisor for group workers becomes for me a matter of conversing in metaphors. By generating images of the social work action in the words we describe, both worker and supervisor come to a mutuality around tasks to be completed in each session and in the work in general. Students and supervisees tend to shy away from the conflict of the group's transition into middle stages, seeing conflict as a sign that the activity is not going well. Metaphors help ground the student in the here and now and open doors of understanding the importance of waiting out silences, amplifying messages and reaching for feelings. With a metaphor in hand, the student enters the group, not with a prescription of how to act, but a broader, more global image to perceive in the action of the group. Movement through the stages of group development with their attendant tasks requires shifts of focus and responsibility for the group facilitator. Metaphors that help identify the stage of group development help students shift focus to move group development ahead in their work. Answering the question of the student "how do I . . .?" with a view through metaphor allows students to discover their own answers in the context of the group, increasing both their feelings of competence but also improving the value of their groups to members. The metaphor relieves students from having a "right answer" to every conceivable situation before attempting to use the group to solve problems and decreasing anxiety about the activity of members.

A student shared about two members of her girls' group who decided that they didn't want to participate in the activity of the group unless it was "what they wanted to do." The group was deciding weekly activities democratically, and, since these girls weren't the natural leaders of the group, their ideas were not being considered by the other members. Trying to repair the group from these "striking" members, the student used a supervisory session to explore possible responses, worrying that she wasn't being successful with the group if all the members were not participating. In supervision we discussed the idea that the two "on-strike" children were like rocks in mid-stream and that the group was going on without their input. The two were working hard to maintain their positions, hoping that by blocking the group's unanimity that might influence the whole. But the group, like water, rushed around them and eventually wore them into joining in with the group's final project, a "movie" of their own making.

Remembering, metaphorically, that water works around obstacles and moves what it cannot wear away, helped my student leave the situation alone so that it could be resolved by the members. Rather than "rescuing" the on-strike girls, the student's ability to maintain the dual focus of democratic process *and* inclusion of all members eventually led to the other members confronting the on-strike girls, reminding them of their important group tasks and finally encouraging them to work on the project that would need all of the members to be completed. The worker indicated that the inclusion that the other members offered the girls was far more than the worker could have engendered by forcing the group to comply with the two members' wishes.

Group middle stages also provide many opportunities to involve the use of metaphors for social group work practice. Members begin jockeying for control and affirmation from other group members. The responsibility of the leader to facilitate the democratic process in the group opens up many opportunities for learning, both for the social work student and for the group itself. In the same way that the life of the group reflects the lives of the members, middles becomes the time that conflicts from outside the group begin to be expressed in the group's process. Providing metaphors to students at this phase of group development offers them a lens with which to see the group's activity.

Members of this same girls' group were also dealing with issues of expectations being placed on them by their families, their schools and by one another in group. Natural leaders had arisen in the group and those members, over and over, were being asked to make group decisions for the others. Whenever the group was confronted with "what to do," all of the members would look to the same girl week after week for her decision, which then became the group decision. If another child offered a suggestion it would only be adopted if the leader approved. Despite efforts at inclusion and asking for additional feedback, the student found members falling back on either the authority of the student herself, or on the natural group leaders to make their group decisions.

Members needed to be challenged to take on responsible roles in the group. The student questioned her decision to ask them to change how they were operating, wondering if she were challenging their self determination by doing so. In supervision we used a metaphor that water needs to be funneled and directed in order to do work. Work within the group becomes another way that new strengths are discovered and new roles are forged. Our discussions included the idea that the pattern in group is like many patterns in their lives, wherein they have other people making decisions for them. As older children, yet not teenagers, they had the terrifying task of developing a sense of what they wanted and expressing it in ways that helped them meet their needs. Rather than take the risk of choosing, the members were colluding to not choose. "Water seeks its own level" was one metaphor that came to mind.

Members were not as anxious to be in charge as they led one to believe by their statements. The reality for them in the group and in life was that they secretly preferred others to decide, while needing to learn how to decide as a point of personal development. The student was able, using these two ideas, to continue insisting that members decide each week on activities and that each week they include all members in their planning. The metaphor allowed her to recognize that the changes would not happen immediately and that the challenges she placed before the group would need to be there a while, creating pools and eddies in the stream of this process until the course would change.

It also reminded us both that to help the group make changes like these, demands for the group's work would have to happen not just once but many times. The change we were asking of them in the middles work was a developmental change. The movement we were asking was from a child's point of view to one of an adolescent. The reluctance to change was born of the crisis they were involved in every day with their families and friends and would not be resolved in one group's lifetime. Use of the metaphors for the work allowed the student to see the group's responses in the context of the group and in the context of their lives and brought new meaning to the "demand" she was placing on them. This allowed the student to continue to encourage the developmental growth that was necessary for this group and to discover the vitality of group for spurring young people to discover their own way of being through normative process.

When teaching group, or talking about it with peers, I find myself constantly drawn to the power of the metaphor as a teaching tool. The use of metaphors makes some very complex behavior more understandable because metaphors tend to not reduce complexity to prescription. Many of my co-workers speak of their reluctance to engage groups because they don't feel prepared to deal with the multi-faceted issues the group brings to the intervention. Metaphors help leaders look at the action of the group in whole measures rather than in discrete events and in this way maximizes the worker's sense of recognition of the group's work while at the same time maintaining their responsibility for the group's continuing development.

I share my first group experience here to say that the metaphors we choose are important to the success we will feel as we apply our social work with groups. It is not enough to simply pick convenient images and to allow them to guide practice. My penchant for water images is born out of my own experiences in groups. When first learning social group work, I was struck by the leader's responsibility to scan the group and to reach for group responses as a means to promote the group's development. This activity was counter-intuitive to every skill I had previously developed. And it was then, as a student myself, that I saw the potential of the metaphor for learning group work. I was reminded that water moves with every touch, either a little or a lot. It has great potential for change of the world around it and it is itself constantly in flux. Cumulative effects make for powerful currents and actions and reactions are affected at every level, both on the surface and deep beneath. As a metaphor for the activities in group, water provides me with an elegant natural model to describe how a change might happen or the way an intervention will be perceived.

Water reminds the student to watch not just the water, but also the shore and to see the subtle response of the world to its presence. No comment or phrase is lost or wasted in group and the water image instructs the student to allow the thoughts and feelings waves to come and crest, to fall and break on the sand of the others, returning again and again as the group defines problems, airs perceptions and reacts to both the leader and the members' responses and completes its work. It is in teaching through metaphor that I find myself able to help students and other social workers feel the wonder at the group's power to transform the human spirit that I feel. You may be thinking about how to encourage students to apply social group work principles to their groups or to make group work understandable to those who have not had the opportunity to run groups in the past. You may be searching for a way to communicate to them the skills you would use. When I am searching for an answer I start with metaphor to make the whole understandable. For myself, I simply remember that group work *is* all wet. And so, I advise my students to dive right in, the water is just fine.

with a male co-leader. I fell into working as co-leader in this situation because I knew about group work and had consulted with him in his beginning work with groups. He was new to social work and group work. For the second group he suggested that it would be easier all round if I literally joined him in the group so that we could work together. In this way he could learn first hand by observing my interventions. It made sense to me to try this approach since, after all, observing and being observed was one of the more useful reasons I understood for co-leading a group.

Without giving any thought to the nature of the group nor to the fact that I would be the only female in a group of men who had been physically abusive to their female partners, I proceeded with the plan thinking that I had the group skills and he had knowledge about the male group members. I would focus on group process, he on the content. It didn't turn out to be that simple. I was so overwhelmed in the beginning as the only female in the room. After the first group session my co-leader told me how surprised he was at my being so quiet and relatively inactive. This was far different from my consultation with him earlier where I was full of suggestions and demonstrated the need to be actively involved in setting the right norms and values for the group, particularly in the early stages of group development. I shared with him how I had felt totally overwhelmed and somewhat frozen, as if by some other force that I felt but could not identify. I had never been in a room with just men, twelve of them, all very uncomfortable with a female being in the room. There had been no preparation for this reaction. I felt their desire not to have me in the room. Neither of us had even considered the impact of gender differences on ourselves nor the group. This population already had difficulty with women and we had not even considered this factor. Inexperience and lack of preparation can truly provide some very surprising reactions.

In retrospect, after co-leading a few groups together, we could look back and identify all that we had discovered and learned about the complexity of co-leadership. We began to debrief after every group session and plan and strategize for the next one. We agreed that it would be necessary to video tape each session in order to have objective feedback about how we were impacting on the group as a whole. Our experiences were different because of gender and the fact that I was the only female in the group and part of a powerful sub-system with ascribed power. We realized that we did not know how to signal each other in the group. We then identified ways we could be in constant communication with each other, e.g., maintaining frequent eye contact by always sitting directly opposite each other. We also coined a few phrases that would be cues to us such as . . . "I was wondering if it would be more useful to . . ." With time and experience the communication between us became second nature. We even learned to strategically discuss in front of the group a decision about group process for the purpose of modeling for them how to negotiate differences, for example. . . (female co-leader) "I am aware of time and think that we might go back to discussing the expectations of the homework for the week" . . . (male co-leader) "I know it's important to do so but I feel that we need to just ask the group what the theme was from the group discussion of the last 15 minutes" (female co-leader) "Then could the discussion be kept to 5 minutes?" (male co-leader) "For sure."

The myths of co-leadership quickly become very evident once I started to co-lead. Some of the myths are: it's very easy for two people to share the work, one can rest while the other works, it is too expensive, and one group leader can achieve the same work. Given that I have worked singularly and with co-leaders, I would say they are very different experiences requiring different preparation. Co-leadership requires a lot of preparation time. The co-leaders must be able to learn how to co-ordinate and synchronize their different styles and approaches for the benefit of the group. For example, I was co-leading a group with a nurse. I was using the social group work model while she was very individually oriented. I would always look to engage the group as a whole, whereas she would have a one on one discussion in front of the group. We had to look at these differences and at least agree that we would try to balance them in the group. I kept trying to teach her about the importance of seeing the group as an entity onto itself that needed to be considered above an individual. I do believe that I did influence her somewhat when she once pointed out to me how aware she was of her training being so individually focused.

Another example of co-coordinating differences lies in a situation where I remember working with a co-leader who tended to be more quiet and less ready to intervene to redirect group process. I was the energetic one who would jump into process without hesitation if necessary. So when it came to one particular group where there was a group member who did not listen to others and could go on for the whole group time about her problems in life completely unaware of anything said to her, we decided that I was the more likely one to intervene firmly to redirect her or bring other members to respond to the theme in her content. In this way we were able to complement our differences for the sake of the group.

Co-leaders must establish a way to communicate to each other during the group sessions that does not disrupt the group process. I remember a time when we as co-leaders had not discussed how to communicate with each other during the group when one of us felt it was necessary to move out of a situation and shift gears for the sake of a group norm or value that was not being addressed. Noticing that my co-leader was being sidetracked from the real issue in the group I suggested to my co-leader that perhaps we could ask the other members about their observations as to what was happening in the group. I had noticed a lot of fidgeting and some members looking as if they were in their own world. The group is a good barometer, particularly through body language, for reflecting to the leadership that an important process in group is being missed. I was aghast when my co-leader said "no" to me in front of the group, that it was important to finish the present discussion. Needless to say after group we had a rather lively debate. The word "no" had left me feeling insulted and undermined. It led to a useful discussion of what words could be a trigger for upset for us individually. We did come to an understanding of how to signal each other when we felt that a particular theoretical concept important to developing a good group process was at stake.

STAGES OF GROUP DEVELOPMENT,
POWER AND CONTROL:
THE BIGGEST CHALLENGE

In one particular group, my co-leader and I were waiting for some of the usual signs that indicated we were "storming," e.g., a member or two would like to split us up as the good vs. bad leader, or the issue of smoking would be raised even though by now it was very common to keep smoking outside of the building, or a ten minute break would be dragged out for double the time. We were starting to believe that we were going to have an exception to the rule, we would jump from Pre-affiliation to Intimacy without going through Power and Control. In reviewing our videotapes of the group sessions it finally dawned on us that we had been duped. Humor had been the form of resistance used. Since laughter is catchy and enjoyable, it camouflaged the challenge to us in a very creative way. This discovery re-invigorated us and moved us as a co-leadership team to a deeper level of understanding of yet more ways that this stage of group development can happen.

I am reminded of another example of getting unexpected outside help to help us move through this challenging stage. It happened in an adolescent group I was co-leading. The school had agreed to provide food for a snack for this group, which was called the Girls' Club. This in itself was quite a big deal and the girls were impressed by this. We had noticed that the girls attacked the food (some for sure had not eaten that day) before all of them had even arrived. We knew that we had to introduce and uphold the value of equality and equal access. As we were both taking turns to suggest to the girls that perhaps they could identify some rules about food distribution, one of the girls picked up a piece of cheese and whipped it at a girl who was standing outside the door ready to enter. What we didn't know was that the principal was walking by and saw the flying piece of cheese. She came into the room and asked what was going on. Her entry totally surprised us all. It was obvious that a long stare was being directed at my co-leader and I. We quickly explained that this was a most unusual circumstance and a few of the girls jumped in and agreed. I am sure that all of us equally being caught by surprise changed their need to rebel against us. The experience of the principal walking in had made all of us simultaneously experience the norms of equality and equal status through our common response. We had no further delay in their all agreeing that the food would be distributed equally once it was clear that everyone who was coming to the group had arrived. We did remember slinking out of the school after the group and discussing outside of the school near our cars whether or not we should even take this incident up with the principal. We agreed that she had far too many worries to deal with than a piece of cheese.

I believe that co-leaders must do the best job they can together for the sake of the group, but as this is not always easy it is then important to do the least damage.

I am reminded of an interagency group program in which my co-leader was assigned to me and I didn't have a say in this. To make matters worse, we were not given much time to discuss our joint work. She felt she was clear about what she had to do as a leader and I was free to do what I felt was necessary in the group and that would be just fine with her, given her overloaded schedule. As the group program progressed I felt that the group was being short changed because we were not working together to model effective inter-communication for the group. I tried to point out to her that we needed to look at was happening in the group. I did not feel heard and regrettably gave up pursuing my point. I had not had an experience so far where I felt that I could not influence or openly discuss group process. I am not sure that the members noticed much of the tension between my co-leader and I because I decided that I would back down and let her take the lead more often than not, for the sake of putting the group ahead of our differences and salvaging what was possible to make this experience a good one.

After that experience I was not prepared to let a program agenda override my, now stronger, belief that co-leaders needed to understand each other and build a way that they could work together. Regardless of the time limitations, I am now convinced that it is necessary to set up a baseline from which to start the process of learning how to communicate effectively. I also now believe that for co-leadership to work it is necessary for two people to be committed to running the group. The investment of time and effort has to be as if it were more than one group.

EDUCATING ADMINISTRATION

It is often necessary, from my experience, to inform and educate agency administration about the complexities and benefits of co-leadership. That was the case regarding the population of women who experienced physical abuse from their male partner or with men who have abused their female partners. The agency was focused on the cost effectiveness of two group leaders and was arguing for one leader per group. I remember strategizing with the other group leaders as to how to explain the need for co-leadership teams. We had to counter a lot of the myths that exist out there, as mentioned earlier. At the beginning we were united in refusing to do groups alone. We were working with populations that had safety issues. We were also looking at the toll it takes to work with these populations. Co-leadership provided an opportunity to debrief, strategize, learn, and consider safety issues with each other about the situations that could occur.

In one of the men's groups, despite assessing the appropriateness of each group member, we would occasionally miss and allow in a member who was inappropriate. One fellow, in particular, was so hostile that if "looks could kill" he would have been successful. We expected anger, but this was far greater anger than we had expected. In fact when we felt and saw that the male group members were fearful of this member, we knew we had to do something. We agonized about what to do and tried different strategies for two sessions. At one point he got very angry with me, even though he was not being addressed personally, and stood up. My co-leader was about to call the police. Even the other male group members had physically shrunk away from him. The body language in the room was clear: Everyone was afraid. We had discussed the possibility that the police might have to be called or the warning made to maintain control. My co-leader, in an ever so quiet but firm voice, told him to sit down and refrain from further discussion because it was clear that he was working himself up into a rage and that was unacceptable in this group. He obeyed. Shaking inside, we finished the group. It took us two hours to calm down and strategize for the next group. We were definitely pulling him out of the group. Group process would not happen if safety was not established. We were the subgroup with the power and obligation to provide safety for the group and proceeded to do so. It was because of the co-leadership team that safety could be dealt with, both for the group and for the co-leadership itself. This incident validated for us the need to teach administration about the necessity of co-leadership for safety and support reasons.

I remember after co-leading women's group for a few years together that we were so in sync that we started to even dress alike. We would show up at group wearing the same sweater or the same color theme in our clothing. We would joke about this with our group and tell them we were in uniform. Our good feelings and comfort created a relaxed atmosphere for the group. This "in sync" behavior reflected to us how deep our level of understanding had progressed as a co-leadership team.

TRUSTING THE GROUP

I have learned that the group begins from the time the first group member is inducted into the group. Trusting that theoretical concepts work and that the co-leaders can apply these concepts effectively takes courage. This brings to mind a particular adolescent girls' group that I co-led in a high school. Working with the girls was a very demanding task, keeping the group leaders constantly flexible and creative. The girls in this group were very boisterous and active. One session, about half way into the group program, one girl brought a video tape of the censored cuts from the Jerry Springer show. She told the group that since it was borrowed she would have to return it the next day and she knew they would all be interested in seeing it. My co-leader and I were stunned. It was against our better judgment to use this time to view this tape. However, we also believed we had to uphold their right to set the agenda and thus the value of democratic process. We also feared that the principal might drop by because she had informed us that she would like to do so at some time within the next few weeks. Sure enough, she did come by. To our horror we heard a knock on the door and knew who it was most likely to be. My co-worker quickly stepped outside and told the principal that this was particularly not a good time to meet with the girls.

In the meantime I am sure we were more shocked than the girls at what we saw on the video. In fact, I found that I had to concentrate on keeping my mouth shut for it would drop open from disbelief. The discussion that followed the video confirmed that we had made the right decision. The girls were able to see how staged and unrealistic this show was. After the group ended and the girls had left we closed the door and burst out in laughter and giggles with the release of all the tension we had felt. We both felt like teenage girls who had almost been caught and got away with it; but we had upheld our beliefs in group process.

Working with adolescents is always challenging. I believe that co-leadership is a requirement for survival in these groups, as well as for maintaining openness and flexibility.

SUMMARY

In summary I can say my co-leadership experiences were truly adventures in learning, growth, and development, both in my skills as a co-leader and as a person.

I have learned many things; however I believe that a few aspects are fundamental for an effective co-leadership team to develop. I've learned that it is important to work as a co-leader with someone you feel is open to learning and struggling with you; who is prepared to see the two of you as a team on a continuum leading to deeper learning and skill development. Taking the risk to be open and honest in communicating is necessary. A good sense of humor has to be a given.

Secondly, I know a co-leadership team needs to advocate for itself with administration for the right amount of time required to properly debrief and plan for each group session.

Thirdly, the social group work model, with its values, norms, and stages of group development, is truly one of the best models from which to work.

Fourth, I discovered that certain populations will be far more challenging than others in what I had to discover about the use of myself as co-leader than I expected, e.g., the adolescents, the all male group.

Fifth, good co-leadership requires that both leaders work a lot before, during, and after each group session.

I now prefer to work with a co-worker with a few conditions being met: that we are on the same wave length, that we can harness our differences in a creative way, and that we can laugh and enjoy ourselves along the way. A lot of work is implicit in all of this.

Reflections on Dealing
with Group Member's Testing of My Authority:
Oy Vey

Alex Gitterman

In reflecting on what influenced my responses to group members'
testing of my professional authority, two experiences immediately
came to mind. First, experiences in my own family significantly shaped
my orientation to authority. As an only child, my energies were devoted
to working out a relationship with my parents. I guess I was spared the
struggle of sibling rivalry. The more I think about it, the more I realize
that my parents were major socializers on how I deal with power, authority, and influence. My parents were very loving and supportive, but
their styles in placing limits and making demands were quite different.
My father conveyed a quiet strength and expressed disapproval gently;
my mother was more intense in setting limits and in demanding respect
and responsible behavior. Without thinking about it, I now realize that I
have internalized both of their qualities in my orientation to authority;
namely, to provide support and simultaneously to make demands initially softly and subsequently more intensely. A second influence was a
high school basketball coach who gained team members' total attention
and unconditional respect. He spoke quietly, never raised his voice, but
firmly communicated his expectations. A stare was sufficient to gain
one's attention.

With these role models and six summers of day camp experiences, I
approached my first year social work placement in a settlement house

[Haworth co-indexing entry note]: "Reflections on Dealing with Group Member's Testing of My Author-
ity: Oy Vey." Gitterman, Alex. Co-published simultaneously in Social Work with Groups (The Haworth Social Work Practice Press, an imprint of The Haworth Press, Inc.) Vol. 25, No. 1/2, 2002, pp. 185-192; and:
Stories Celebrating Group Work: It's Not Always Easy to Sit on Your Mouth (ed: Roselle Kurland. and Andrew
Malekoff) The Haworth Social Work Practice Press, an imprint of The Haworth Press, Inc., 2002, pp. 185-192.
Single or multiple copies of this article are available for a fee from The Haworth Document Delivery Service
[1-800-HAWORTH, 9:00 a.m. - 5:00 p.m. (EST). E-mail address: getinfo@haworthpressinc.com].

185

with relative confidence. My assignments included work with a group of youngsters, ages 10-11, and a group of adolescent boys. Despite my prior experiences in working with latency aged children and pre-adolescents, the adolescent group was going more smoothly than the younger group. The adolescents' testing of my authority was relatively benign. I remember, for example, as the ending of the first meeting approached, the group informed me of a ritual for evaluating new leaders. They would thump on the table and then on signal place their thumbs in an upward motion signifying approval or a downward motion signifying disapproval. In this ritual, the worker also had to evaluate his performance. When the moment came to reveal the direction of thumbs, my thumb was the only one in the upward position. The notion that I was the sole person to approve of my performance struck me as so funny that I could not stop laughing. The members joined me in uncontrollable laughter. Then, they informed me that this was actually a test to see how a new leader would react to a negative vote. My convulsive laughter met their test, as the ability to laugh at oneself was essential to their normative system. Later, the members engaged in more complicated testing, like sneaking alcohol into an agency dance, but members were always willing to work on the underlying issues. With these youngsters, spontaneity, consistency, and caring carried the day.

In contrast, I was more attuned to applying my newly learned social work skills with the younger group. When the boys were unruly, I stated in my softest professional, bland voice, "I see that you are upset today." And when they knocked chairs over and uncontrollably ran around the room, I would "skillfully" comment, "I see you had a bad day in school today." The calmer I remained, the wilder the members became. At that time I did not realize that my words and emotions lacked congruence. The discrepancy between words and emotions made members progressively more anxious and intensified their acting out behavior. One afternoon the indigenous group leader decided to "help" me with the discrepancy between content and affect by hitting me hard on the back of my head. He must have realized that it would take something drastic and dramatic to get this neophyte's attention and to spur him into action.

Well, it worked! All my newly learned social work skills went out the window as I grabbed this youngster and picked him up and in a very non social work response yelled, "Fuck this–don't you ever, I mean ever, put your hands on me or anyone else in this group." The other youngsters exclaimed, "Ooh, ooh Al is mad, Al is mad." I yelled for all the boys to sit down and firmly stated, "I am sorry for cursing and yelling, but this shit is going to stop–no more throwing chairs–no more hitting each other. From this day on we are going to show respect for each other and learn to get along." From that moment on the group coalesced, the work began and a new and totally unexpected level of mutual aid evolved.

The youngsters had been testing my authority and begging for greater structure and limits; my inability to deal with the testing made them very uneasy. They were also unnerved in not knowing what might happen once I lost my cool–would I hit them, desert them, etc. They saw me at my worst–a flash of anger, followed by a congruent message–. . . "I will take charge and this will be a safe place for all of us–I may get mad, but I still will care about you and want to help you." They finally received what they wanted from me: greater structure and congruence. They taught me an important lesson about integrating verbal and non-verbal, about creating structure for freedom of expression and for making demands and showing caring that were mutually inclusive rather than exclusive.

After graduating from school, I worked as a gang worker and youth program director. I continued to struggle with issues related to testing of authority. However, the testing processes became even more intense and confusing as I began my first experience in working with African/American youth. Lacking the experiential base for understanding the Black experience in America and the functions served by testing of authority, I personalized their reactions and vacillated from feelings of hurt and rejection to feelings of despair and resignation. I was not prepared for the intensity of their pain, for the intensity of their resentment, and for the incessant demand that I prove myself as worthy of trust. A persistent testing of rules, peer rivalries, and crises left me drained.

I had a reoccurring dream that I was African/American and hoped that magically the adolescents would come to accept and trust me. What I did not realize was that the act of testing is in itself an act of engagement. The youngsters had to care about me to invest themselves in building a trusting relationship. Indifference and withdrawal were the foe rather than active testing. While their challenges threatened my professional self-esteem, these youngsters were teaching me a powerful lesson about meaningful relationships–they had to be earned and they had to be worked on. Their message was that people could care about adults without verbalizing the caring and that it could be expressed in unexpected and unpredictable ways.

I vividly remember, for example, playing basketball in the playground with a group of tough, really tough, teens. A youngster ran out of the projects with great angst and informed us that President Kennedy had been assassinated. At that very moment, the boys spontaneously made a circle around me to protect me from potential harm. And I had doubted their caring! When I left the agency, it was the youngsters who had given me the most difficult times (broken my car antenna, let the air out of my tires, put sugar into my gas tank) who also invited me to their weddings, funerals for family members and friends, and sent birth announcements. They were wonderful teachers about the testing of authority, dealing with interpersonal obstacles and reaching across racial and developmental barriers.

In my next position as director of a settlement house, I was very fortunate to take a seminar for new field instructors with William Schwartz. He introduced me to brand new group work concepts and literature. An article by Bennis and Sheppard (1956) particularly caught my attention. I was struck by the powerful notion that group interpersonal processes were significantly affected by stages of group development. The authors conceptualized what I experienced in practice, namely that as a group begins and throughout its life, members work out their relationship to the worker and to each other. The authors taught me that the initial phase of group life was characterized by a preoccupation with the worker's authority. Testing of the worker's authority (its consistency, fairness, boundaries) was a normative process and essential to group life. Before members could turn their energies toward each other and develop interpersonal trust and intimacy, they had to become less preoccupied with the worker and testing his/her authority. These ideas "spoke to me" and placed my prior practice experiences into a schema.

As an agency director and subsequently as a faculty field instructor of a unit of students, I saw the relevance of these ideas outside of group life. Testing of authority was also inherent in the role of administrator, supervisor and field instructor. With the new concepts in hand, I dealt with the testing processes very differently. They were depersonalized–they were not about me, but rather about improving the quality of our relationship. This new perspective was fully tested during my first teaching experience. In the Spring of 1968, I was invited to teach an introductory group work course for non majors at an urban graduate school. Before teaching my first class, I was fortunate to have read Garland, Jones, and Kolodny's (1968) brand new and powerful article on the stages of group development. The authors conceptualized and illustrated a sequence of five stages of group development that progressed from pre-affiliation, power and control, intimacy, differentiation to separation.

The class for non-majors was composed of second year students, thirteen majoring in community organization (two-thirds male) and eleven majoring in casework (four-fifths female). The community organization students were significantly more active in class discussions than the casework students. Many had prior experiences in the Peace Corps and Vista Volunteer programs. Also, the female casework students permitted the male community organization students to dominate class discussions. The community organization students were more sophisticated in their socio-political perspectives, but the casework students had greater curiosity about and identification with professional methods and skills. One group had greater vision; the other group had greater interpersonal skills. One group shouted; the other group reflected. I visualized the class as composed of members from two divergent professions.

The teaching challenge was to find the common ground and create a climate where the community organization students would engage the casework students in broadening their social vision and, in turn, the casework students would engage the community organization students in increasing their interpersonal skills. After a brief honeymoon, I found myself struggling with the community organization students to move beyond the '60s slogans and to become more interested in turning vision into professional skills. The casework students were receptive to viewing their clients through broader theoretical lenses. I made the mistake of dealing with the community organizing students' challenges by over "selling" my ideas. The class (an early one) ended with a strong power struggle. In the subsequent class, only the casework students participated. About a half-hour into the class I realized that the community organization students had organized a "silence strike." After a moment of intense anxiety, Bennis and Sheppard and Garland, Jones, and Kolodny entered my consciousness. I visibly relaxed and thanks to these authors a potential threat was experienced as an exciting opportunity.

I suggested that the community organization students' silence spoke loudly and invited them to share their concerns. They remained silent. I said that I had been so busy with trying to convince them of my ideas about professional function that I was not listening and respecting their professional traditions and viewpoints. I continued that I was "all sold out" and ready to listen and that now it was their turn. After a brief silence, the community organization students voiced their objections. Interestingly, the conversation also empowered the casework students. They paralleled the community organization students' complaints about my not respecting their traditions with how they experienced the attitudes of the community organization students toward them–that they did not appreciate being referred to as "junior shrinks." This dialogue led us to examine our historical professional roots and divergent professional traditions. We finally were listening to and learning from each other. I now viewed the community organization students and their silence protest as my allies in moving our work forward rather than as a threat to my professional self-esteem. I no longer repeated my earlier mistakes.

I would like to describe one additional practice experience that revealed a different and unexpected type of testing of authority. On my first sabbatical I wanted the experience of working with a group of adolescent girls and volunteered in a suburban high school. I collaborated with the director of social work to compose a group of sophomore and juniors who were dealing with loss. During the first meeting, the director introduced me as Dr. Gitterman. This created an immediate distance between the girls and me. Was I a psychiatrist and did that mean that the school identified the girls as having mental health problems? Understandably, they were uncomfortable and cautious with me. At the same time, working with adolescent girls was a new experience for me and I was uncomfortable with their giggling, miniskirts, etc. We felt ill at ease with each other.

The first two meetings were characterized by silences, awkwardness and gossiping among the members. I had never expected that this experience would be more difficult than working with gangs. At the third meeting, a member, with the support of others, tested my willingness to join the group's interpersonal system by asking me to share a happy and a painful life experience. I was struck that they were not testing my authority but rather my willingness to be intimate. This was my first clue that gender differences might affect group stage theory. At that moment, the group was coalescing to test my willingness to "belong" to the group. I was amazed at the creativity of their challenge: "You have to be personal and intimate with us before we will speak personally to you." I had to earn their intimacy. I had to model openness and sharing that I wanted them to do with each other and with me. If my response had been, "We are here to discuss your troubles and not for me to answer personal questions," I would have put up a metaphoric wall and the members would have withdrawn from the experience. The members responded to my sharing of a happy experience as well as a painful loss by sharing their own losses (death of a parent, divorce, etc.). At that moment some moving, focused and intense work began. Responding to the member's question in a genuine and non-defensive manner represented a turning point in the group's life as the members turned away from their preoccupation with me toward helping each other with their life issues.

As I look back on earlier practice experiences, how much the stage models of group development would have helped me and, later, did help me with group members who tested my authority strikes me. I end my essay with further reflections on the concept of a stage model. Initially, the stage models' prescriptiveness and linearity provided some logic and order to what I often experienced as an unpredictable and unorderly group process. As my practice experiences became more diverse, I increasingly realized that the prescriptiveness and linearity of the stage models were its major strengths, but also a significant limitation. For example, the girls' group challenged my willingness to be intimate and not my authority, as the model would predict. I made the mistake of fitting a group experience into a model rather than being curious about its applicability for diverse group populations in different agencies and environments (Berman-Rossi, 1992, 1993; Kelly and Berman-Rossi, 1999; Schiller, 1995, 1997).

I now question whether the issue is to further refine a stage model of group development or make a paradigm shift. Group process is different when the agency has power over group members' lives rather than functioning as a benign or malevolent force. Group process is different when the group is composed of angry male adolescents as compared to female survivors of sexual abuse. Group process is different when the worker and group members differ in backgrounds. Group process is different based on the degree or lack of homogeneity in group composition. Group processes, like life itself, are phasic. These processes ebb and flow in response to the interplay of group members and the environment. Stages of group development separate group processes into distinct stages that are not really distinct in actual practice.

I agree with Schwartz (1971, p. 9) that the interplay of two factors, the worker's authority and members' interpersonal relationships, "provides much of the driving force of the group experience." But I find that these forces do not appear in sequential stages. Rather authority and intimacy themes are always present. Sometimes they appear together in the foreground; other times one moves into the foreground and the other recedes into the background. These movements are not fixed or linear, but rather transactional and are influenced by such factors as culture, race, ethnicity, socio-economic status, gender, social cohorts, sexual orientation, and agency context.

REFERENCES

Bennis, W. and Sheppard, H. (1956). A theory of group development. *Human Relations.* 9: 415-37.

Berman-Rossi, T. (1993). The tasks and skills of the social worker across stages of group development. *Social Work with Groups.* 16 (1/2): 69-92.

Berman-Rossi, T. (1992). Empowering groups through understanding stages of group development. *Social Work with Groups.* 15 (2/3): 239-255.

Garland, J., Jones, H., and Kolodny, R. (1968). A model of stages of development in social group work groups. In S. Bernstein, (Ed.). *Explorations in Group Work*, pp. 12-53. Boston: Boston University School of Social Work.

Kelly, T. and Berman-Rossi, T. (1999). Advancing stages of group development theory: The case of institutionalized older persons. *Social Work with Groups* (22): 2/3, 119-138.

Schiller, L. Y. (1997). Rethinking stages of development in women's groups. *Social Work with Groups.* 20 (3): 3-19.

Schiller, L. Y. (1995). Stages of development in women's groups: A relational model. In R. Kurland and R. Salmon, (Eds.). *Group work practice in a troubled society*, pp. 117-138. New York: The Haworth Press, Inc.

Schwartz, W. (1971). On the uses of groups in social work practice. In W. Schwartz and S. Zalba, (Eds). *The practice of group work*, pp. 3-24. New York: Columbia University Press.

Creating a Group Work Culture in a Children's Mental Health Agency: A Professional Memoir

Marion S. Levine

Since 1974, I have served as the executive director/CEO of the North Shore Child and Family Guidance Center (NSC&FGC). NSC&FGC is a major children, adolescent, and family based mental health service on Long Island. It provides a wide array of therapy, educational and training programs that reaches thousands of residents each year. Its professional staff members are primarily a mix of social workers, psychologists and psychiatrists. The agency has struggled to stay solvent, autonomous and innovative.

The case I make for its present dynamism, in spite of years of serious government budget cuts (cuts that have laid low other community mental health services), is that the survival and success of this organization is rooted in its origins. Lay and staff relations were interdependent. Neither side dominated the other in their respective roles. This made it easier for me to extend a style of leadership which heavily utilized social group work principles and practices.

LOOKING BACK:
A DANCING TEACHER'S TALE

My entry into the field of social group work started with the convergence of unexpected events. Like many young women in the 1950s, be-

---

[Haworth co-indexing entry note]: "Creating a Group Work Culture in a Children's Mental Health Agency: A Professional Memoir." Levine, Marion S. Co-published simultaneously in *Social Work with Groups* (The Haworth Social Work Practice Press, an imprint of The Haworth Press, Inc.) Vol. 25, No. 1/2, 2002, pp. 193-202; and: *Stories Celebrating Group Work: It's Not Always Easy to Sit on Your Mouth* (ed: Roselle Kurland, and Andrew Malekoff) The Haworth Social Work Practice Press, an imprint of The Haworth Press, Inc., 2002, pp. 193-202. Single or multiple copies of this article are available for a fee from The Haworth Document Delivery Service [1-800-HAWORTH, 9:00 a.m. - 5:00 p.m. (EST). E-mail address: getinfo@haworthpressinc.com].

193

ing a good student meant to me that maybe I could also be a good teacher. I gravitated, as many others of my generation did, into a major in education at Brooklyn College.

Despite the low tuition I needed some living expenses. Financial support from home was not easily forthcoming. My mother was a widow and not particularly sympathetic to college education for girls. She thought I should enter the job market. But I knew that I needed some money to make my way through my school years without burdening my family.

My then-boyfriend had already established himself as a children's and youth worker in the Brownsville section of Brooklyn. He had befriended the social workers who ran the Brownsville YM-YWHA. He thought that I had the right personality to work with children. His recommendation and my good performance at an interview landed me a part-time beginner's job. I was literally assigned to be a "gatekeeper." This experience, combined with my growing impatience with a very stilted education curriculum at Brooklyn College, was to be the impetus for my entry into the field of social work.

My first job as gatekeeper was an odd one, but it turned out to be a good opportunity to test my talents. The Brownsville "Y" was located in a second floor loft in a so called "changing neighborhood." There had been many disruptive incidents and the administration of the "Y" wanted someone to screen members before they entered the building. In my isolated post on the first floor, I became what amounted to a respite worker for children having difficulty fitting in on the second floor, where most of the programs took place.

Within a few months I was making a noticeable impression on my bosses. I remember particularly being lauded for taking a very depressed African American eight-year-old girl under my wing and bringing her out of her doldrums and into a successful group experience (a forecast, I think, of my later second career as a psychiatric social worker).

My supervisors were MSW social group workers from the best graduate schools. They were very impressive role models. I was soon to be allowed to lead groups and be formally supervised by them in "the group process," a miracle to me.

Meanwhile, I had to go through some preliminary steps. I was promoted to game-room worker. The game room was a serious problem area. Chaos resigned. The children would arrive full of restless energy from a day of sitting in school. They ran wildly in circles. I remember picking up a jump rope and funneling their running in my direction into an unending contest of high jumps. I intuitively realized that the rope organized the running. The activity corners that I soon set up were also just the cue needed to engage different youngsters with the diversion of their desires. I was catching on to how one structured an informal setting and was succeeding at it.

To round out my experience, and to earn a few extra dollars, I accepted a challenge from a nearby agency, the Brownsville Boy's Club (BBC). I was asked, "How about taking over their teenage lounge on Wednesday nights?" They wanted to see if I could tame the "wild beasts." Not all of these teenagers fit the description, but some did. They were made up of one part social wallflowers, one part genuine juvenile delinquents, one part budding basketball stars and one part good boys with bad influences surrounding them.

I would teach them all social dancing. They would check their weapons at the door, utter no profanities during the evening and behave like gentlemen. They would be dancing with "Hooker's" girlfriend. Hooker was the nickname of my husband to be. He had been the president of the 2000 member club, was a very popular and respected figure in the neighborhood, a long time boy staffer at the BBC.

The experience with the dance club was extraordinary. The natural structure of teaching and learning to dance and the skill needed to perform well was just what many of these so called "tough boys" needed. The fact that they were learning to relate to "girls" from Hooker's girl was both titillating and esteem-building for them. It was widely noted that Wednesday night, "the night Marion taught the group to dance," was practically the only evening when there never was a fight or a disruptive incident at the club.

I discovered that it was indeed true, as I had been told by others, that I did have some natural talent in directing activities in both informal and formal group settings. I was on my way into the profession of my lifetime, most of which has been spent in the field of children's mental health.

CULTIVATING A GROUP WORK CULTURE

North Shore Child and Family Guidance Center's 1950s beginnings were rooted in a community based model where progressive minded suburban activists organized to establish a children's mental health clinic for less affluent members of the community. These lay leaders hired social work and psychiatric staff who offered a high quality professional service, albeit a rather traditional brand of individually-oriented therapy for children and counseling for parents. Many community educational activities were also provided.

A dual governing structure grew up. First came the North Shore Child Guidance Association. These were the lay volunteers who were responsible for building and maintaining a geographically representative chapter movement, raising a modest sum of money through fund-raising events and carrying out a widespread educational program about mental health issues. The North Shore Child Guidance Center, the other unit, was the professionally directed clinic. The word "Family" was added to the name in the '80s to reflect the reality of our treatment and program practices.

When I arrived as executive director in 1974, I proceeded (with the aid of a handful of staff members who had some training in group work) to vastly expand the use of groups in the agency. This meant not only enlarging the number of community education groups and professional training groups, but also a big expansion of group therapy and support groups. Previously, therapists referred their patients to groups that were seen largely as ancillary, as a socialization enhancer but not necessarily as a primary therapeutic experience.

Group supervision was widely utilized. Staff teams were organized to carry out diagnostic, treatment, planning and administrative functions. Key administrators met with me to hammer out consensus decisions in groups where maximum participation was encouraged. This change called for a new emphasis in our staff development program. Much more training in skills for leading or utilizing groups was offered.

On the board and volunteer level, a major transformation was also taking place. In the '50s and '60s, volunteer activities and organizational leadership was " a woman's thing." By the 1970s, work and professional opportunities were vastly changing the lives of the suburban women whose efforts built and maintained our organization. While there was still a very dynamic remnant in the leadership group, there was less energy in the chapter movement. The chapter movement slowly declined and a more centralized leadership organization evolved. While women still dominated, a significant number of male leaders were recruited and soon served in top spots.

New board structures also followed the large-scale expansion of fund raising that the board authorized. This was unlike the other free-standing community mental health centers on Long Island, whose budgets were almost exclusively dominated by government contracts and fees. A bruising fight against a hospital takeover of the agency finally collapsed in 1975. This struggle proved to be a red light. A conscious desire to maintain a high level of autonomy in the face of erratic government support animated the board's willingness to take on difficult financial tasks. They began to accept the need to do far more fund raising than previously.

To make this happen, program advisory groups, long range planning groups, financial development groups, and the like were formed. Board development and the recruitment of new members representing philanthropic, business, political and multi-ethnic elites became priorities.

Board and volunteer involvement was most successful when highly planned presentation and discussion processes were put together. Attention to good group dynamics became paramount. Intentional planning for these processes became an administrative staff challenge that was not taken lightly.

Along with the expanded use of groups in the internal administration of the agency, the art of coalition building was crucial to success when we created joint enterprises with other organizations (many from the fields of education and health). These alliances added to our ability to access funds other than through mental health streams. We could expand our reach and still stave off pressures from hospitals to merge or pressure on us to take over smaller agencies whose cultures we found to be incompatible to our own. We preferred short-term cooperative ventures. We worked to reduce bureaucratic and competitive power factors. Single programmatic purposes dominated these relationships. Much emphasis was put on the diplomatic training of our staff leaders who engaged in these joint ventures. Managing the inevitable group conflicts that naturally emerged was given a high priority in the staff's skills acquisition.

Changing demographics in the Long Island suburbs also deeply influenced the kind of client who came to our doors and the form of therapy we recommended. This resulted in the need for a growing cultural sensitivity on the part of our staff and for special cultural competency training. We initiated an aggressive outreach approach to reach racial and ethnic minorities.

This often called for setting up highly visible and concrete services, such as our Hispanic Family Life Project, our Haitian Immigrant Project and many black oriented programs such as Good Beginning for Babies. Strong signals were given that we were there with culturally relevant services, many of which were of a group work nature.

As we developed new facilities, we made sure that they were accessible to the broadest group of Long Islanders. In addition to minority groups and new immigrants, much larger numbers of working and lower middle class white ethnic families came to our doors. The reduction of stigma in seeking help for emotional problems and the reduced influence of church-dominated counseling brought our numbers up among this population.

Our low fees for service, our no waiting lists and our increased referral and marketing approaches also broke down resistance in many diverse client groups.

The makeup of our staff also changed rather dramatically. "People of color diversity" and white ethnic diversity grew among our professional and support staff. These new staff members came to be even a longer percentage of the whole than the previously dominant numbers of Jewish and WASP professionals.

STAFF DEVELOPMENT

The mix of staff members was also characterized by large ratios of social workers to psychologists and psychiatrists. While social workers were more likely to be sympathetic to the use of group related practices than the other professions in our agency, this was only marginally true. By the 1970s there was already a visible reduction in the number of group workers who were in therapeutic positions in mental health agencies. The practice mode of social work therapists on staff differed only slightly from that of the other individually oriented psychotherapists who dominated our psychology and psychiatry departments.

Given a chance to acquire new skills, many casework-oriented social workers did react positively to staff development workshops in group work. Some still resisted, but others saw it as a professional enhancement. Still this was going against the grain. The pattern for social workers in mental health settings had been to take additional postgraduate training at psychoanalytic institutes. Many of our staff members did this. This was, as many of us remember, the real ticket to professional growth and development. This absorption left little time or desire for the acquisition of group work skills.

REACHING OUT

To further announce that we were a leading center for group work practice, under the leadership of Andrew Malekoff, who is presently our Associate Director, we created the Long Island Institute for Group Work with Children and Youth.

This unit enhanced our prestige as a training center for professionals and non-professionals in a variety of youth serving agencies. A survey that the Institute conducted among hundreds of these workers showed conclusively that the overwhelming number felt that they lacked the skills to make them successful in leading groups. They agreed that they needed more training. The Institute also has sponsored periodic region-wide conferences on group work practice.

We also launched a number of special projects which became particular employment magnets for recently trained social group workers, many from the Hunter College School of Social Work. Perhaps the best illustration of the intensity of the use of the group work model is the highly innovative Intensive Support Program (ISP). This school-based mental health collaboration between North Shore Child and Family Guidance and Nassau Board of Cooperative Educational Services (BOCES) has become a model program for helping youngsters with serious emotional disturbances.

The goal is to maintain these students in the least restrictive, most inclusionary environment through an intensive support program. It aims to improve academic and social/emotional adjustment of these students while reducing the costs of caring for them by preventing long-term residential placements. Presently in its fifth year, ISP has grown from a small program to a huge multi-site initiative.

ISP's stated goal is to build on the strengths of the students. It seeks to help them by supporting the development of positive family communication, by creating a caring school climate, promoting safety at home and in school, and by having clear rules and consequences for behavior. It emphasizes constructive use of time in school and at home. In addition to individual and group therapy, there are many examples of special group work activities that promote the students' positive assets. They are illustrated in detail here because it has become rare in school settings or in therapeutic settings to make such extensive use of activity groups for the seriously emotionally disabled child or adolescent. The use of these activity groups, which came naturally in our practice when some of us began our careers, has now become atypical. At ISP we now sponsor the following groups. They represent a return to activity groups led by a trained social worker and remind me of my early days in the Brownsville Boys' Club.

- Art stock 2001–in its third year. It is a showcase for students' talents in painting, sculpture, ceramics, poetry, and music.
- Poetry Club–Part of the elementary school ISP program, it offers enriched opportunities for self-expression through the written word.
- Self Expression through Movement–Here we link communication of the student's interior life with body movement.
- Relaxation Exercise Groups–Students draw upon their own inner resources to achieve a more peaceful state.
- Real Life Group–Elementary students improve their understanding and mastery of every day challenges, with visits to such places as supermarkets, post offices, and railroad stations.
- Career Readiness Project–A special Youth Employment staff is deployed; one of its aims is to familiarize students with the interview process. Mock interviews with members of the business community as preparation for the real thing are offered.

SEPTEMBER 11th, 2001

The terrorist attack on New York on 9/11/01 provides a final note on how the norms of North Shore Child and Family Guidance have become dependent on our ability to effectively gather people into intentional and purposeful groups.

Our first response to 9/11 was to bring our entire professional and support staff together on the day of the attack to both reorganize our services to meet the new emergency and to reassure them that the agency was there to support them to deal with their own shock and fear.

We went on a twenty-four hour/seven day alert. As a result of the rapidity of our response and the special units we deployed to deal with trauma and bereavement, we soon became important to many client groups, such as surviving spouses and their families, schools and their staffs, corporations, and community and religious groups. Grief-related support groups were created across the age spectrum. Hundreds were served in the immediate aftermath of the tragic event. Comprehensive services are planned for the future anticipation of post traumatic stress and other psychologically delayed effects.

Our annual Board of Directors/staff strategic planning meeting had been scheduled for the evening of 9/11. We rescheduled for a month later. We decided that business as usual was not in order. Instead, we devised a group process that encouraged that participants would share how 9/11 had affected them personally as well as its impact on their roles as board and staff members.

Our board members, who were used to routine business meetings, reported gratitude at the opportunity to share and connect with each other in a moment of great stress. It was proof again, they said, that their dedication to the Center had not only great benefit to the community but to themselves as well. Some called the experience a defining moment for themselves and for the organization. This kind of testimonial to the magic of a good group process is something all of us in the field hear often.

Risking and trusting the group process at moments of crisis was the right thing to do. My faith in first principles, combined with a well developed personal stubborn streak, provided the needed strength to fight off many destructive fads and fashions that came along every few years. I considered them dangerous and alien incursions into our profession. We all know them well. They included the push to adopt business models, medical models, prescriptive psychotherapy models, and the most dangerous and most seductive of them all, becoming over-dependent on outside forces, which I call "the government as the ultimate sugar daddy" model.

Adopting one or another of these models might have done us in. Saying no was often very difficult. "That's the only way to go," many said. But we resisted. The result is that we're not only still standing but in the opinion of others, we're thriving.

FULL CIRCLE

My early experiences in social group work with difficult children and youth taught me well not to make assumptions about what is or isn't possible, in even the most dire circumstances. I learned to enter a situation with openness. Willingness to do almost anything necessary to prevail was combined, in my mind and heart, with a conceptual value-based position that believed passionately in the use of non-authoritarian practices. I discovered that this way of thinking and acting can take you far. I learned, as we all would, that our children want to do their own thing as well as be given a context in which to do something well. It was this series of part-time jobs working with kids in Brownsville that became the groundwork for my work with groups and individuals in a social work career that has now spanned almost 40 years.

I was well taught by the immediacy of the situation and by the vitality of the groups in these poor neighborhoods. I learned to reach for strengths, for the potential in children and youth and their parents, and to respect and value the power of the group process.

T - #0535 - 101024 - C0 - 212/152/12 - PB - 9780789017475 - Gloss Lamination